The Ultimate Obamacare Handbook

The Ultimate Obamacare Handbook

(2015–2016 Edition)

A Definitive Guide to The Benefits, Rights, Responsibilities, and Potential Pitfalls of the Affordable Care Act

Kimberly Amadeo

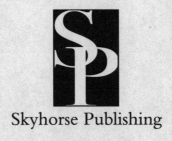

Skyhorse Publishing

Skyhorse Publishing books may be purchased in bulk at special discounts for sales promotion, corporate gifts, fund-raising, or educational purposes. Special editions can also be created to specifications. For details, contact the Special Sales Department, Skyhorse Publishing, 307 West 36th Street, 11th Floor, New York, NY 10018 or info@skyhorsepublishing.com.

Skyhorse® and Skyhorse Publishing® are registered trademarks of Skyhorse Publishing, Inc.®, a Delaware corporation.

Visit our website at www.skyhorsepublishing.com.

10 9 8 7 6 5 4 3 2 1

Library of Congress Cataloging-in-Publication Data is available on file.

Cover design by Rain Saukas

ISBN: 978-1-63450-561-1
Ebook ISBN: 978-1-5107-0155-7

Printed in Canada

Table of Contents

Table of Contents

INTRODUCTION

You need facts, not opinions, and this handbook delivers just that. This book is based on extensive research done using credible sources and real-life interviews with people who have personally been helped by the Patient Protection and Affordable Care Act (more commonly called the Affordable Care Act or Obamacare).

The Ultimate Obamacare Handbook gives you resources you can use, like:

- A guide to how health insurance works.
- Step-by-step instructions to signing up for insurance.
- Descriptions of various tax exemptions.
- Definitions of the key terms used in the Affordable Care Act (ACA), health insurance, and health care.

You'll also find out how Obamacare has been quietly improving the lives of Americans since it was signed in 2010. For example, 100 million people received free preventive care. They got their chronic diseases treated before they needed to use expensive emergency room services. That has *already* lowered costs, not only for them but for everyone.

You'll learn things like why mandatory coverage is needed for the benefits of the ACA to work. You'll be introduced to real people who have already been helped. (Disclaimer: Although the stories are all true, most of the names and identifying information have been changed to protect their privacy.)

Most importantly, you'll understand how the ACA affects you specifically and the steps you can take now to make sure you're getting all the benefits you deserve.

How to Use This Book

I strongly advise you to read the entire book from cover to cover. That's the best way to understand Obamacare. This book clarifies it all. In chapter 1, you will learn how Obamacare was created and, more importantly, who really drove the reform. You'll uncover the real reason why Obamacare was needed in chapter 2. In chapters 3 and 5, you'll learn about all the benefits that you already receive, even without doing anything. The ten essential benefits are in also in chapter 5.

To really understand health insurance, how it works, and why America relies on it, read chapter 4. If you're curious about why the mandate was needed, that's in chapter 8. Benefits for seniors, small businesses, and charities are explained in chapter 9. These chapters give you all the information about how the ACA affects you, your family members, and your community.

You can also start with the chapters that apply to your immediate situation. They are organized so you can refer to the ones you most need at the moment. If you are looking for basics, like how to get insurance, go right to chapter 6. That's where you'll also find whether you're exempt from Obamacare's mandate. Read chapter 7 to find out whether you qualify for a subsidy. Taxes are in chapter 10. Definitions of the most important Obamacare terms are at the end of the book in How to Speak Obamacare.

This book is designed to be used as a handy reference. You can carry it with you when you go to the doctor, meet with an insurance broker, or even watch the news. You can quickly find the information you want anytime you need to get up to speed.

The Patient Protection and Affordable Care Act is the biggest law since Social Security. The publishers and I want this to be a positive, useful book for you. We've seen how it has helped, and hurt, our families and friends. Now we want to empower you to make your own decisions based on how the law affects not just segments of society, but you and the people you care about the most.

Chapter 1

WHAT IS OBAMACARE?

Most people think of Obamacare as simply the health insurance offered on the Health-care.gov website, but it's a whole lot more. Obamacare is actually two federal laws. The Patient Protection and Affordable Care Act (Public Law 111-148) was signed into law on March 23, 2010, while the Health Care and Education Reconciliation Act (Public Law 111-152) was signed seven days later.

The Truth About Obamacare

There are a lot of misconceptions about what Obamacare does and doesn't do. Answer the following questions to test your knowledge.

True or False?   The Affordable Care Act is much better than Obamacare.

False, since they are the same thing. However, 45 percent of Americans polled in a 2012 Gallup survey approved of the ACA, while only 38 percent approved of Obamacare.[1]

True or False?   A majority of Americans want Obamacare to be repealed.

Not exactly. It *is* true that more than half (54 percent) of Americans are opposed to Obamacare. However, they don't all agree it should be repealed.

- 35 percent are opposed because it's too liberal. They are the ones who want it repealed.
- 16 percent think it's too conservative. They're opposed because it doesn't go far enough in providing affordable health care, but they don't want it repealed.
- 12 percent are opposed only because they think the Act has *already* been repealed.
- 7 percent think it was overturned by the Supreme Court.[2]

True or False? Health insurance costs are rising because of Obamacare.

True and false. The true part is that health insurance premiums have been rising. For example, average premiums for company-sponsored family plans rose 4.8 percent a year from 2005 to 2010. Since the ACA was passed, premiums increased at a slower rate—3.8 percent a year.

Privately-bought plans were worse, averaging from 15 percent to 20 percent premium increases before Obamacare. Once the exchanges opened, the subsidy affected price increases in both directions. A 2014 Kaiser survey found that 46 percent of those who switched from a privately-bought plan to a subsidized plan saw their premium payments drop, while 39 percent were hit with an increase.[3]

The "false" part is that health insurance costs were rising, but not because of Obamacare. For the truth behind health insurance costs, see chapter 4. In addition, the plans available now have more benefits thanks to the ACA, so obviously they would cost more. These benefits are described later in this chapter in the section "Summary of the PPACA."

True or False? If you like your plan, you can keep your plan, period. President Obama said this right from the beginning. He meant that the ACA itself had no provisions that canceled anyone's plan. In fact, it had a provision that helped many keep their plans. Many plans that were in place before the ACA was passed could be "grandfathered in," if they met some minimum requirements.

Mostly false. Many people still lost their plans for a variety of reasons. Some companies found it was cheaper to pay the penalty than continue offering health insurance. They knew their employees could find cheaper plans on the exchanges. One million people had plans that didn't comply with the ACA's requirements, and so their insurance companies dropped them.[4]

Many "grandfathered-in" plans were dropped by the insurance companies anyway. In 2014, Kaiser Permanente canceled policies for 3,414 customers in Maryland and Virginia. Humana did the same for 6,544 policies in Kentucky. Many companies simply decided it didn't make business sense to maintain such a wide variety of plans at different costs.[5]

True or False? Obamacare intrudes into the doctor-patient relationship. Government bureaucrats will decide your treatment, not your doctor.

Partly true, except this hasn't really changed with Obamacare. Your doctor decides on the treatment, but an insurance company staff person decides whether the treatment will be covered, how much will be covered, and how much the doctor will be paid for it. If it's a very expensive treatment, and the insurance won't pay for it, the doctor may change to a similar treatment that is covered or let you self-pay. The only time the government is involved in this decision is when it acts as the insurance provider with Medicare and Medicaid. The relationship between doctor and patient really hasn't changed with the ACA.

True or False? Obamacare cuts benefits for those on Medicare.

False, although 44 percent of people believe it's true. That's because the ACA cuts funding for Medicare by $716 billion over ten years. The cuts affect providers in the following three areas:

1. Hospitals receive $260 billion less because they'll switch from fee-for-service to value-based care. That means you'll receive more follow-up care after leaving the hospital. For more on that, see chapter 3.
2. Insurance companies that provide Medicare Advantage plans receive $156 billion less. That's because those plans cost the government 17 percent more than regular Medicare for the same services in 2010. The ACA now limits cost increases so they will be closer to regular Medicare costs.[6]
3. Home health care, skilled nursing services, and hospice receive the rest of the cuts. For more on who pays for Obamacare, see chapter 10.

Most people don't know that the ACA increased the number of actual benefits Medicare recipients receive. They now get free preventive care like physicals and mammograms. They will eventually receive 75 percent funding for the Part D "donut hole" prescription drug costs. The donut hole refers to the gap in coverage that began once Kimberly: Awkward $2,860 was spent that year on meds (in 2011). After that, seniors paid 100 percent until they hit a ceiling, at which point Medicare picked up its share again. For more on how the donut hole is being phased out, see chapter 9.

True or False?   All your personal and medical information will be combined into a giant database so the government can keep better track of you.

Mostly false, but here's why people believe it. First, you provide personal information to the health exchange when you apply for an insurance plan. It might feel a little creepy, because the application on the exchange asks for your Social Security number; your income from your last tax statement, paystub, or W-2 form; and personal data, like whether you smoke and the ages of you and your children. This information is needed so the IRS can check it against its records to make sure you qualify for any subsidy. That means the IRS pretty much has all this data anyway. The question about smoking helps determine what your premiums will be since health insurance companies are allowed to charge more for smokers. If this seems unfair, read chapter 2 and you'll find smokers are much more likely to get lung diseases such as cancer and COPD (Chronic Obstructive Pulmonary Disorder).

Second, the ACA pushes the medical profession into using computerized health records. Going forward, your medical information will be moved from filing cabinets to a computer database. Theoretically, that could one day be connected to the data on the exchanges, but it hasn't happened yet. It's still being set up, and that project is challenging enough.

Could a despot one day use all this computerized information to control your life? Probably, but there is already so much data about you, and everyone else, on computer servers and clouds that the ACA doesn't represent a serious new threat to your privacy. In other words, don't avoid getting the subsidy on the health exchanges because you're worried about "Big Brother." If you have a Social Security number, pay taxes, and use credit cards, your privacy is already compromised.

True or False?   Obamacare is socialized medicine, similar to health care in Canada or Great Britain.

Nearly completely false, although 57 percent of Americans think it's true. In Great Britain, the doctors are employees of the federal government. In Canada, the government pays most medical bills. The Canadian system is similar to the one the United States already has with Medicare and Medicaid. The ACA does expand Medicaid, so in that particular case you could accurately make the argument that it's promoting socialized medicine. The rest of the ACA expands the private insurance market.

People may be confused because President Obama's initial proposal was to extend to the rest of us the health coverage Congress enjoyed. That coverage is a Medicare-like program where the government pays the bills. Congress rejected this proposal in favor of the current plan, which relies on private health insurers.

Ironically, Obamacare took the members of Congress, and their staff, off of their Medicare-like program and forced them onto the private exchange, just like everyone else. In that case, the ACA actually reduced socialized medicine.[7]

True or False? Under Obamacare, you're forced to pay higher premiums for services you don't need, such as pregnancy, childbirth, and maternity care.

Mostly false. No matter what kind of insurance you get, you're paying for services you don't need and hopefully never will. For example, if you're a fitness buff, you're paying for diabetes services you'll never need. Women pay for prostate tests they'll never need, and so on. Auto insurance allows some customizing, such as windshield breakage, but most states require a minimum coverage to protect the general good of the public. And that's the purpose of the pregnancy, childbirth, and maternity coverage mandated by the ACA. For reasons why, see chapter 5.

True or False? Obamacare establishes "death panels" that allow the government to make decisions about end-of-life care for people on Medicare.

False, although 40 percent of people believe it does. In 2009, former Alaska Governor Sarah Palin posted on Facebook that the ACA created "death panels" that determined whether Medicare recipients would receive funding to extend their life, or whether they should just go into hospice.[8]

She misunderstood the actual ACA provision. It would have instructed Medicare to provide 100 percent free coverage for doctor appointments with recipients who wanted to discuss do-not-resuscitate orders, end-of-life directives, and living wills. Thanks to the controversy surrounding her statement, the provision was dropped. However, in 2015 the CMS revived the idea of paying doctors to hold advance-planning conversations with their patients.

True or False? My tax dollars pay for illegal immigrants to get health insurance from Obamacare at a discount.

Mostly false. The ACA prohibits illegal immigrants from obtaining health insurance on the exchanges. However, anyone can get preventive care at community health centers. Payment is on a sliding-fee scale based on income. The ACA expanded community health center services to treat those who currently rely on expensive emergency rooms as their primary health centers. To find out why you really do want illegal immigrants to get free health care, see chapter 5.

True or False? By offering free childbirth coverage, Obamacare creates incentives for illegal immigrants to come to the United States so their children will be American citizens. These so-called anchor babies then make it easier for the parents to become citizens themselves.

Somewhat true. Illegal immigrants cannot get Medicaid or Obamacare insurance. However, the 1986 federal Emergency Medical Treatment and Labor Act (EMTALA) requires hospitals to treat anyone who shows up in the emergency room. Medicaid already refunds around $2 billion a year to hospitals that treat at least 100,000 illegal immigrants. Half of the funds go to California hospitals alone. Medicaid does not fund prenatal care. For more, see chapter 4.

Does this create an incentive for illegal immigrants to give birth in the United States? The statistics say probably not, and here's why. The $2 billion a year spent by Medicaid has remained pretty stable throughout the years. If it were an incentive, it would have increased during the recession. Instead, there were actually fewer illegal immigrants then. This means that the primary motivation for immigration is jobs, not free citizenship.[9]

True or False? Businesses aren't hiring because of Obamacare and uncertainty over its regulations.

Mostly false. The requirement to provide insurance only affects a tiny number of companies. That's because businesses with fewer than fifty employees are exempt from the requirement. They compose 5.8 million out of the six million companies in America.

Although they provide most (65 percent) of all *new* jobs, they only employ thirty-four million out of the one hundred forty-six million *existing* workers.

What about the two hundred thousand companies with more than fifty employees? Most of them aren't really affected because 95.9 percent already offered insurance before the law even took effect. Of those companies, only 10 percent said they were reducing their workforce, cutting hours, or hiring more part-time, temporary or contract workers. Since most of these companies already offered insurance, the cuts and reductions are probably not because of the mandate. They're more likely part of a cost-cutting trend caused by the Great Recession.[10]

True or False? The ACA will create "Taxmageddon," a massive tax increase of $800 billion over the next ten years. This is the largest tax increase in US history.

True-ish. Obamacare tax increases will take in $76.8 billion a year when they are all up and running in 2018. This is the highest amount of any tax increase in history, and these taxes do slow economic growth right when it's trying to recover from the recession.

Although this is the highest amount, the next tax increase is right behind it. The 1993 deficit reduction bill increased taxes $65.9 billion a year. However, that comparison doesn't take into account inflation, population growth, income growth, and economic growth. You really should look at tax increases as part of a bigger picture.

For example, if you take into account inflation, then the 1982 tax increase was the largest, collecting a whopping $85.3 billion in today's dollars. If you compare the tax increase as a percent of the total economy, then the 1942 tax increase to fund World War II was the largest—it was 5.04 percent of total economic output, compared to just 0.43 percent for the ACA.[11]

Media Negativity Means You Might Be Missing Benefits

Don't feel bad if you didn't do as well on the quiz as you thought you would. Since 2010, you've been bombarded with fifteen times more negative than positive news about the Affordable Care Act.

Since the law was passed, $445 million has been spent on ads, according to Kantar Media CMAG. Guess how much was anti-Obamacare? A whopping $418 million, which funded 880,000 ads that attacked the Act. Most of these were local ads centered on supporting state and congressional political campaigns.

Only $27 million went toward the fifty-eight thousand ads that were positive. Another $700 million was spent by the federal government to help you sign up on the exchanges. That isn't counted as positive advertising because it's not designed to counter the negative articles. It simply explains how and why you must sign up if you don't already have insurance.[12]

As a result, there is a lot of misinformation about the Affordable Care Act. Most of the criticism focuses on how it takes from the middle class and gives to the poor.

Others point out that it's just a tool President Barack Obama and the Democrats use to buy votes. For example, a 2012 *Forbes* article reports that half of American households receive either Medicaid, food stamps, Medicare, Social Security, or unemployment compensation. The writer argues that Obamacare's expansion of these entitlement programs means that a majority of Americans will vote for whoever promises to keep sending those checks. Meanwhile, he says, taxes keep rising on businesses and hardworking middle-class Americans who must support those on the government dole. He adds that this discourages the entrepreneurship and free-market system that makes our economy the strongest on earth.[13]

A few argue that the ACA is basically unconstitutional and moves America away from its core values, taking us another step closer to socialism and a new world order. Most people have made up their minds about the Affordable Care Act based on this debate.

It's no wonder that so many people have a negative opinion of Obamacare. A 2013 poll by the Urban Institute found that nearly 41 percent had an unfavorable view.

However, what you don't know about Obamacare *can* hurt you. You could be missing out on benefits as a result. For example, of those who had an unfavorable view:

- **Almost half (43.3 percent) qualified for subsidies**. By being opposed to the ACA, they were leaving money on the table.

- **Nearly a third (31.3 percent) were uninsured.** These are the very people Obamacare was designed to help. Did they prefer taking their chances of winding up with an enormous emergency room bill and going bankrupt as a result?
- **More than 44 percent had incomes that were too high to benefit from subsidies, and/or had insurance already.** They probably didn't think Obamacare would help them. They didn't realize how wrong they were. The ACA helps everyone by lowering healthcare and Medicare costs and improving the quality of hospital care, as explained in chapter 3.
- **Over 29 percent of those who were opposed were on Medicaid or another public health plan.** Why would they be against something that made their life better? Perhaps they just didn't want anyone else to get government-subsidized health insurance.
- **Nearly one-third were eligible for Medicaid.** Many didn't even know it and were missing out on crucial health care they could have gotten for free.[14]

Some people are opposed to the principle of government getting involved in health insurance even when they could benefit from it. And good for them for sticking to their values.[15]

However, most probably don't know how they benefit or understand how they can take advantage of the plan. If you're one of them, this book is for you.

The point is that negative media portrayals of Obamacare keep many of you from getting the benefits you deserve. That's right, 10.7 million Americans qualified for insurance subsidies, didn't realize it, and didn't apply for coverage on the health insurance exchanges. If Obamacare is repealed, you can lose benefits you already have that you don't even know are from the ACA.

Ironically, most people like what the ACA does; they just don't like Obamacare. The Kaiser Family Foundation found that 88 percent of people surveyed like that small businesses can get tax credits to buy insurance for their workers. Only 52 percent know that's because of Obamacare. Again, 81 percent love that Medicare is paying for more of the cost of the "donut hole" in the prescription drug program. Only 46 percent realize that's thanks to the ACA. Eighty percent like the health insurance exchanges, but only 58 percent know that the Affordable Care Act is responsible.

What *did* everyone know about Obamacare? Around three out of four knew that it mandated big companies to provide health insurance, and 57 percent thought that was a good idea. The same number knew about the individual mandate, but only 40 percent approved of it.[16]

Summary of the Patient Protection and Affordable Care Act

Can you understand Obamacare without reading all 2,572 pages of the entire law that enacts the Affordable Care Act? Absolutely. That's because it's already laid out in ten easy-to-summarize sections called titles. The implementation of the Act falls under the Department of Health and Human Services (HHS), except for Titles VIII and IX, which are managed by the Treasury Department.

Below is a summary of each of the ten titles and what they actually do.

Title I. Quality, Affordable Health Care for All Americans. This is the most important and familiar title. It's the section that requires every American citizen to have insurance or pay a tax. However, subsequent regulations provide exemptions for many Americans. Title I sets up the health insurance exchanges. It authorizes federal funding for state exchanges while allowing the federal government to run the exchanges if needed.

This title requires businesses with fifty or more employees to provide health insurance or pay an excise tax. A subsequent regulation delayed this requirement until January 2015 to give businesses time to gear up. The title allows companies with fewer than 100 employees to use the exchanges. It provides tax credits to small businesses (twenty-five employees or fewer) that offer insurance and provides subsidies to businesses that offer health insurance to early retirees aged fifty-five to sixty-four.

Title I also requires insurance companies to provide these popular and critical benefits, which are covered in more detail in chapter 5:

- Parents can add children up to age twenty-six to their plans.
- Companies can't deny coverage to those with preexisting conditions (children in 2010, adults in 2014).
- Companies can't drop people if they get really sick.
- Plans cannot put a limit on either annual or lifetime coverage.
- Plans must cover 100 percent of wellness, pregnancy exams, and other preventive procedures.
- Insurance companies must spend at least 80 percent of premiums on medical services, or rebate the rest back to policyholders. They must submit justification for rate hikes to states for approval.

Title I requires that all insurance plans provide some services to address each of ten essential benefit categories. It's up to the states and insurance companies to define exactly what services will be included. The first seven boost preventive services. They include wellness exams; maternity, newborn and pediatric care; prescription drugs and lab tests; and mental health. These are designed to treat illnesses before they require a trip to the emergency room. The three remaining benefit categories include those that are covered by nearly all health plans, including emergency and hospital care. You'll find more details, and how this lowers health-care costs, in chapter 5.[17]

Title II. The Role of Public Programs. This title expands Medicaid coverage to those earning 138 percent or less of the federal poverty level. It guarantees coverage for adults without children for the first time ever. It also extends coverage for foster-care children until they turn twenty-six. It funds 100 percent of the expansion for the first three years, and 90 percent after that.

It expands the Children's Health Insurance Program (CHIP), which allows states to add health benefits for children that are greater than the standard Medicaid benefits. The average income level for families receiving CHIP is 241 percent of the poverty level, much higher than for Medicaid. States can opt to increase coverage up to the level of their state employees' plan, standard Blue Cross and Blue Shield plans offered to federal employees, or a standard HMO plan.

Title II gives the states $40 million to promote enrollment of both Medicaid and CHIP. That's because nearly five million uninsured children were eligible for the programs but were not enrolled.[18]

Title III. Improving the Quality and Efficiency of Health Care. This title helps Medicare beneficiaries by closing the "donut hole" in Medicare Part D prescription drug coverage. It also requires that all insurance plans cover 100 percent of wellness and preventive care visits.

Title IV. Prevention of Chronic Disease and Improving Public Health. Title IV established the National Prevention, Health Promotion, and Public Health Council to support preventive health care. This includes programs to lower cholesterol or blood pressure, lose weight, stop smoking, and control diabetes.

Title V. Health Care Workforce. This title increased public funding to pay for additional primary care physicians, nurses, physician assistants, mental health providers, and dentists.

Title VI. Transparency and Program Integrity. Doctors must report any conflict of interest they have. This occurs if they own or have any other financial interest in labs or other testing facilities and refer patients to them. They must also provide a list of alternative testing facilities to patients. All drug companies and medical supply manufacturers must report any financial arrangements they have with doctors, including any gifts they make. All pharmacy benefit managers for Medicare or exchange insurance plans must report the discounts they negotiate with drug companies. They are encouraged to recommend generic drugs whenever possible.

Title VI also identifies high-risk providers and prevents them from setting up in a different location. It gives states the ability to test legal reforms to enhance patient safety. It prevents elder abuse by providing training to nursing home staff and requiring they undergo background checks.[19]

Title VII. Improving Access to Innovative Medical Therapies. This title funds a drug discount program in hospitals that serve low-income patients. It also requires competitive pricing for vaccines and hormone therapies.

Title VIII. Community Living Assistance Services and Supports Act (CLASS Act). The CLASS Act was the only title that was subsequently found to be unworkable. It was supposed to allow disabled Americans to receive a $50 daily payment to put toward assisted living. They would have had to pay premiums for five years and work for three of those years. The daily payment would go toward home health care, adult day care, and other services that allowed them to stay in their homes. Or the payment could have gone toward assisted living facilities, nursing homes, or group homes.

This title, had it survived, would have been self-funded. It was estimated to reduce the federal deficit by $70.2 billion over the next ten years as it allowed people to keep working and stay out of nursing homes and the hospital. It became effective on January 1, 2011, but by October 1 it was abandoned. Basically, it could not compete with private sector plans that offered better benefits for the same price.[20]

Title IX. Revenue Provisions. This title raises Medicare payroll taxes to 2.35 percent on incomes above $200,000 for individuals or $250,000 per family. These taxpayers pay 3.8 percent Medicare taxes on the lesser of dividends, capital gains, rent, and royalties, or on income above the limits stated. For details on the tax, see chapter 10.

Title X. Reauthorization of the Indian Health Care Improvement Act. Title X modernizes health-care services for 1.9 million Native Americans. It's implemented in consultation with the Indian Health Service.

The Real Architects of Obamacare

Although President Obama is accurately credited with getting health-care reform passed, he didn't do it alone. Many people, including journalist and political commentator Bill Moyers, say that the health insurance industry itself was behind the Affordable Care Act.

It certainly looks that way when you learn who was involved. First, here's some background information. The health insurance industry has six lobbyists for each and every member of Congress. Most lobbyists are former congressional staff members.

Second, the health insurance industry, in trying to ensure that a public option did not survive spent $380 million on lobbying, advertising, and campaign contributions in the three months prior to the ACA being passed. Montana Senator Max Baucus received $1.5 million. He then introduced the bill when he was chairman of the Senate Finance Committee. Another $50 million went to the other members of that Finance Committee.[21]

Senator Baucus's "Chief Operating Officer" was Liz Fowler, who had been WellPoint's (now known as Anthem) Vice-President of Public Policy from 2006 to 2008. While working as the top health adviser for Baucus, she coordinated writing the bill with Obama's staff. Prior to that, she was Baucus's chief health aide from 2001 to 2005.

Baucus's former top health adviser was Michelle Easton, who later became a lobbyist for WellPoint. Another member of Senator Baucus's "Gang of Six" was Republican Senator Mike Enzi. He proposed a similar bill in 2006 that was written by Stephen Northrup, his aide from 2003 to 2006, who then became WellPoint's Vice President of Federal Affairs in 2007. Northrup had written the bill introducing Medicare Part D while Executive Director of the Long Term Care Pharmacy Alliance.

Baucus said he removed the public option, favored by President Obama, because he couldn't get the sixty votes needed to pass it. However, it may be more than a coincidence that he and his team have so many connections to the health insurance industry, which wouldn't benefit from any health-care reform that excluded them.[22]

Physician lobbying groups were also involved. In fact, the American Medical Association (AMA) wanted the ACA to change Medicare's fee-for-service payment system to a bundled payment plan. The AMA felt this would be the same as a pay raise for doctors. This has actually happened. For more on how payments have changed under the ACA, see chapter 3.

The ACA was patterned after a similar program in Massachusetts. Its architect, MIT economist Jonathan Gruber, was another key adviser in drafting the Obamacare bill. In fact, Gruber said both health-care reform measures relied on the "three-legged stool" to make the whole thing work. The first leg was mandated insurance coverage for everyone. This was needed to get the relatively healthy people into the insurance pool. Second, they both ended insurance discrimination against those with preexisting conditions. This would help those with preexisting conditions afford preventive care and keep them out of the hospital emergency rooms and their expensive treatments. Third, they subsidized health insurance for the poor for the same reasons. Together, the goal was to lower health-care costs for everyone, but most importantly for the government.[23]

Another driving force behind Obamacare was Ezekiel Emanuel, the White House special adviser on health policy, and brother to Chief of Staff Rahm Emanuel. His stance on health care in America is one reason there were so many rumors about government intervention in health care and death panels. In a 2007 *Journal of American Medicine* article, Emanuel said a major reason for the rise in health-care costs was expensive medical technologies, drugs, and treatments. For example, one drug that treats metastatic colon cancer extends the average life span only two to five months, but costs $50,000. He argued that insurance companies should only pay for these expensive new treatments when the evidence demonstrates that they work for most patients.

He also argued that the best way to cut health-care costs was to focus spending on adolescents instead of children or the elderly. His reasoning was that society hadn't invested in children yet, but had invested a great deal in educating adolescents. Their potential had yet to be tapped. The elderly, on the other hand, had already produced most of what they had to give to society and so shouldn't be the top priority when distributing scarce economic resources. This kind of talk scared many people.[24]

Chapter 1: References

1. Peter Grier, "Obamacare vs. Affordable Care Act: Does the Name Matter?" *USA Today*, November 29, 2013. http://www.csmonitor.com/USA/DC-Decoder/Decoder-Buzz/2013/1129/Obamacare-vs.-Affordable-Care-Act-Does-the-name-matter, accessed October 13, 2014.

2. Kevin Robillard, "Poll Shows 54 Percent Against Obamacare," *Politico*, May 2013. http://www.politico.com/story/2013/05/poll-54-percent-against-obamacare-91902.html, accessed October 13, 2014. "Kaiser Health Tracking Poll: April 2013," The Henry J. Kaiser Family Foundation, April 30, 2013. http://kff.org/health-reform/poll-finding/kaiser-health-tracking-poll-april-2013/, accessed October 13, 2014.

3. Robert Farley and Lori Robertson, "Obama Mixing and Matching Insurance Stats," FactCheck.org, March 18, 2014. http://www.factcheck.org/2014/03/obama-mixing-and-matching-insurance-stats/, accessed October 14, 2014. Liz Hamel et. al., "Survey of Non-Group Health Insurance Enrollees," Kaiser Family Foundation, June 19, 2014. http://kff.org/private-insurance/report/survey-of-non-group-health-insurance-enrollees/, accessed October 14, 2014.

4. Tom Cohen, "Debunking Four Obamacare Myths: Both Sides Get It Wrong," CNN.com, November 5, 2013. http://www.cnn.com/2013/11/05/politics/obamacare-debunking-myths/, accessed October 11, 2014.

5. Louise Radnofsky and Anna Wilde Mathews, "Some Insurers Cancel Plans," *Wall Street Journal*, October 3, 2014.

6. Sarah Kliff, "Romney's Right: Obamacare Cuts Medicare by $716 Billion. Here's How," *Washington Post*, August 14, 2012. http://www.washingtonpost.com/blogs/wonkblog/wp/2012/08/14/romneys-right-obamacare-cuts-medicare-by-716-billion-heres-how/, accessed October 13, 2014. "Letter to Honorable John Boehner," Congressional Budget Office, July 24, 2012. "Medicare Advantage Fact Sheet," The Henry J. Kaiser Foundation, May 1, 2014. http://kff.org/medicare/fact-sheet/medicare-advantage-fact-sheet/, accessed October 13, 2014.

7. Tara Culp-Ressler, "Americans Still Have Big Misperceptions About Obamacare," ThinkProgress, March 21, 2013. http://thinkprogress.org/health/2013/03/21/1753731/obamacare-misperceptions-poll/, accessed October 13, 2014. "Members Only," *The*

Wall Street Journal, August 7, 2013. http://www.wsj.com/articles/SB1000142412788 7324522504578654193173779414, accessed October 13, 2014.

8. Jenny Gold, "Poll: Three Years Later, Americans Still Don't Understand Health Law," Kaiser Health News, March 20, 2013. http://khn.org/news/poll-three-years -later-americans-still-dont-understand-health-law/, accessed October 13, 2014.

9. Phil Galewitz, "Medicaid Helps Hospitals Pay for Illegal Immigrants' Care," Kaiser Health News, February 12, 2013. http://www.kaiserhealthnews.org/stories/2013/ february/13/medicaid-illegal-immigrant-emergency-care.aspx, accessed October 11, 2014.

10. Angie Drobnic Holan, "Top 16 Myths About the Health Care Law," PolitiFact.com, September 24, 2013. http://www.politifact.com/truth-o-meter/article/2013/sep/24/ top-16-myths-about-health-care-law/, accessed October 12, 2014.

11. "Biggest Tax Increase in History?" FactCheck.org, July 10, 2012. http://www.factcheck .org/2012/07/biggest-tax-increase-in-history/, accessed October 12, 2014.

12. Carla K. Johnson, "Spending on Negative Obamacare Ads Outpaced Positive Ones Significantly, Study Shows," Associated Press, July 16, 2014.

13. Merrill Matthews, "Seven Things (Still) Wrong With Obamacare," *Forbes*, July 5, 2012.

14. John Holahan, Genevieve M. Kenney, Michael Karpman, and Ariel Fogel, "Looking Behind Opinion Polling on the Affordable Care Act," *2013 Health Reform Monitoring Survey,* Urban Institute, February 26, 2014. http://hrms.urban.org/briefs/ aca-opinions.html, accessed July 25, 2014.

15. Olga Khazan, "Rich, White, Healthy People Are Most Likely to Hate Obamacare," *Atlantic Monthly*, March 3, 2014. http://www.theatlantic.com/health/archive/ 2014/03/rich-white-healthy-people-are-most-likely-to-hate-obamacare/284149/, accessed July 26, 2014.

16. "Kaiser Health Tracking Poll," Kaiser Family Foundation, March 20, 2013. http://kff.org/health-reform/poll-finding/march-2013-tracking-poll/, accessed July 25, 2014.

17. "Sec. 1302. Essential Health Benefits," PPACA. http://en.wikisource.org/wiki/ Patient_Protection_and_Affordable_Care_Act/Title_I/Subtitle_D/Part_I#SEC. _1302._ESSENTIAL_HEALTH_BENEFITS_REQUIREMENTS, accessed July 29, 2014.

18. "Benefits," Medicaid.gov, http://medicaid.gov/chip/benefits/chip-benefits.html; "Connecting Kids to Coverage," Department of Health and Human Services, 2010. http://www.insurekidsnow.gov/professionals/reports/chipra/2010_annual.pdf, accessed July 29, 2014.

19. "Read the Law: Affordable Care Act Section by Section," US Department of Health and Human Services. http://www.hhs.gov/healthcare/rights/law/index.html, accessed October 12, 2014 "Title VI. Transparency and Program Integrity," WhiteHouse.gov, https://www.whitehouse.gov/health-care-meeting/proposal/titlevi/diclosure-physician-financial-interests.

20. "Health Care Reform and the CLASS Act," Kaiser Family Foundation, April 28, 2010. http://kff.org/health-costs/issue-brief/health-care-reform-and-the-class-act/, accessed October 12, 2014.

21. Bill Moyers, YouTube. https://www.youtube.com/watch?v=hZ5tj4cN9Jk, accessed October 13, 2014.

22. "WellPoint 'Really Did' Write the Baucus Health Plan," *Physicians for a National Health Program*, September 25, 2009. http://www.pnhp.org/news/2009/september/wellpoint_really_di.php, accessed September 28, 2014.

23. "10 Obamacare Questions Answered by MIT Economist Jonathan Gruber," *The Daily Beast*, March 29, 2012. http://www.thedailybeast.com/articles/2012/03/29/10-obamacare-questions-answered-by-mit-economist-jonathan-gruber.html, accessed October 11, 2014.

24. Betsy McCaughey, "Obama's Health Rationer-in-Chief," *Wall Street Journal*, August 27, 2009. http://online.wsj.com/articles/SB100014240529702037066045743744632800986 76, accessed October 11, 2014.

Chapter 2

WHY HEALTH-CARE REFORM WAS OBAMA'S TOP PRIORITY

When President Obama took office in 2009, the United States was in the worst recession since the Great Depression. Millions were out of work, and the financial system had barely recovered from total collapse. However, once he passed the American Recovery and Reinvestment Act of 2009, the new president's next big push was to reform health care. Was this really more important than reforming Wall Street, controlling the debt and deficit, or taking action on global warming? It was, but not for the reasons you might think.

The President stated his case for the ACA in a *New York Times* editorial on August 15, 2009, titled "Why We Need Health Care Reform." He gave the following four ways his reform would "provide more stability and security to every American." His plan would:

1. Provide affordable insurance to those who didn't have it and to those who were tied to a job they didn't like just to get the health benefits.
2. Lower health-care, Medicare, and Medicaid costs by reducing inefficiencies and subsidies to insurance companies.
3. Shift Medicare benefits from insurance companies to seniors, and require Medicare to pay 100 percent for prescription drugs.
4. Offer basic consumer protections to those with preexisting conditions.

You'll notice that his second and third reasons say pretty much the same thing—lower Medicare costs. That tells you something. It sums up the real, underlying reason why health care needed to be reformed—it was taking over the federal budget.

Medical Care Is Uncle Sam's Biggest Expense

In 2010, lawmakers finally passed the ACA to contain the cost of Medicare. That year, the Fiscal Year 2009 budget estimated the cost of Medicare and Medicaid at a whopping $632 billion combined. That's 20.3 percent of the total FY 2009 budgeted spending of $3.107 trillion for just two programs.

What lawmakers disliked was that they could not do anything about this spending in their annual budget process. Once established, programs like Medicare and Medicaid are part of the mandatory budget. That means the amount spent could not be changed without an actual act of Congress. That's because it took an act of Congress to pass them in 1965 during the Johnson Administration. The $632 billion put into the budget was just an estimate of what would be spent. Elected officials could not simply change that amount each year, like they could with the programs in the discretionary budget.

The only budget item in 2009 that was bigger was Social Security, at $644 billion, and it was part of the mandatory budget too. However, it was funded completely by payroll taxes, which show up as FICA on your pay stub. You also have payroll taxes taken out for Medicare, but those taxes only pay about half the total cost of the program.

Reducing health-care costs is a high priority for anyone interested in lowering the US debt. The more Medicare and Medicaid cost, the bigger the deficit. It left even fewer funds for discretionary programs that Congress could control. In fact, by the time all $1.996 trillion in mandatory programs including the interest on the national debt were paid, only 39 percent of the budget was left over for the discretionary budget. And two-thirds of *that* went to defense and related security spending. This only left $482 billion to run everything else in the discretionary budget, including the departments of Justice, Education, Transportation, and Agriculture.

The largest non-defense department in the discretionary budget was HHS. It received $70.4 billion to manage Medicare, Medicaid, and other health-related payments. (Although $70.4 billion is a lot of money, it's still just one-tenth of what was spent on defense and security-related spending like Homeland Security.)[1]

Now, the federal government spends $943.2 billion on health care alone—more than anything else, according to the FY 2015 budget. This includes Medicare benefits ($530 billion), Medicaid benefits ($333 billion), and the HHS, which manages the programs ($80.2 billion). The next largest budget items are Social Security, at $891 billion, and combined military spending, at $732.7 billion. Once you subtract the $229 billion paid for the interest on the national debt, and the rest of the mandatory programs, it only leaves Congress $334.1 billion to run the rest of the federal government.[2]

The problem only gets worse. By 2025, spending for Medicare and Medicaid alone will rise to more than $1.5 trillion. That's $954 billion for Medicare and another $567 billion for Medicaid—and that's just the benefits, not the administration. Thanks to the recession, many Baby Boomers won't have enough saved up for retirement. Sadly, they will need to go on Medicaid because they won't even be able to afford their Medicare co-payments.[3]

Medicare fraud was also on the rise. Some estimates put the cost as high as $60 billion a year. That's money that comes out of taxpayers' pockets and goes directly into the pockets of thieves.

The only way to keep mandatory spending from taking over the budget was to cut the growth of health-care spending. That was the underlying reason Obamacare was proposed and the real reason both the Senate and the House passed it. All the other reasons you've heard are nice-to-haves for portions of the population. The real reason was money and retaining congressional power to spend it.

Politicians have known for years that something had to be done. However, until 2010, circumstances were never right. The Clintons famously failed to pass health-care reform. Bush even worsened the problem by passing Medicare Part D without any funding. However, during Obama's first term, both houses of Congress were controlled by his party. He knew that he might not get another chance to pass such a controversial piece of legislation. His personal priority was to do something about climate change, but the impact of out of control health-care spending on the federal government's budget couldn't wait.

Who Pays for Medicare?

Unlike Social Security, Medicare's payroll taxes and premiums cover only 51 percent of its cost. Additional taxes on Social Security income pay another 2 percent.

The Medicare Hospital Insurance Trust Fund, by investing all prior year's proceeds, covers another 3 percent. Before the ACA, Medicare was projected to run out of money in 2017. The ACA extended its life expectancy by simultaneously increasing taxes and lowering the cost of health care.

The rest of Medicare's costs (43 percent) is paid for by either federal (41 percent) or state (2 percent) contributions. Those expenditures are either covered through higher taxes, or added to the government debt.[4]

There are four parts to Medicare, and each is funded differently. Here's what they are and where they get their money:

Medicare Part A. This is the Original Medicare that President Lyndon B. Johnson established in 1965. It pays for hospital costs. In 2013, its expenses were $251.1 billion. Most of that (88 percent) was paid by payroll taxes. Premiums from people who didn't pay taxes during their career contribute 1 percent. Taxes on Social Security benefits contribute 6 percent. The Medicare Trust Fund pays for 5 percent.

Medicare Part B. This pays for doctor visits. Most of it (73 percent) is paid for by the general fund, which means it contributes to the deficit each year. In 2013, it cost $255 billion. None of the Medicare payroll taxes pay for it. That means 25 percent is paid for by premiums, while just 2 percent is paid for by the Trust Fund.

Medicare Part C. This is the Medicare Advantage program. It's funded completely by the premiums paid to the private insurance companies that manage it.

Medicare Part D. This was added by President George W. Bush in 2003. It pays for prescription drugs. Like Medicare Part B, it contributes to the national deficit, since 77 percent is paid out of the general fund. Fourteen percent is paid by premiums, so that's the only part that pays for itself. Thirteen percent is paid by the states, adding to their deficits.[5]

Where Does the Money Go?

The biggest slice (30 percent) of the Medicare payment pie goes toward hospital costs. That's 24 percent for inpatient care and 6 percent for outpatient services. The next biggest piece (25 percent) goes toward the federal portion of Medicare Advantage Plans.

These are private insurance plans that cover benefits such as vision, dental, and hearing coverage. The federal government also pays private insurance companies to administer Medicare Parts A and B. The remaining Medicare funds go toward doctor visits (12 percent), prescription drugs (11 percent), and nursing homes/home health care (8 percent), with 14 percent spent on miscellaneous services like hospice and dialysis.[6]

Of course, soaring health-care costs affect everyone, not just Congress and its ability to spend. One out of three Americans are having trouble paying their medical bills. Surprisingly, most of them have health insurance, meaning they can't afford their coinsurance, deductibles, and premiums. Others can't pay for bills not covered by their insurance. This debt was accumulated before the Obamacare exchanges were open, so much of it is from those health insurance "loopholes," like annual limits, that the ACA has closed, as discussed in chapter 5.[7]

In 1960, the nation spent just $27.4 billion on health care, or $147 per person. Health care was just 5 percent of total economic output as measured by GDP (Gross Domestic Product). By 1990, it had more than doubled, to 12.2 percent of GDP.

By 2010, health-care spending had risen one hundred times, to $2.6 trillion. That's 18 percent of the nation's economic output, which was the highest percentage in the developed world. The average health-care cost in America was $8,411 per person, twice the amount spent by Europeans, Canadians, Japanese, or Australians.[8]

Since 2010, costs have been rising more slowly, but still faster than the rate of inflation. The Council of Economic Advisors (CEA) projected that if health-care costs kept growing at the same rate, they would eat up one-third of the US economy by 2040. To cut the cost of health-care spending, the ACA needed to address the root causes.

Seven Reasons Why Health Care Costs So Much

Why is US health care so much more expensive than in other developed countries? Below are the seven major reasons:

1. People live longer. Improvements in health care over the last fifty years have done a great job of extending life. Unfortunately, they haven't slowed the aging process. Between 2000 and 2010, the number of people who died from strokes fell by 20 percent.

Sadly, the 6.8 million survivors were severely compromised by paralysis, language problems, and memory loss. This increased the cost of health care, and that trend is expected to only get worse.[9]

As technology advances, it creates increasingly more expensive ways to save lives. For example, as of 2012, more than a third of hospitals were using expensive robotic surgery that hadn't even been invented thirty years earlier.[10]

2. The elderly make up a larger percentage of the population. The seventy-five million Baby Boomers are aging. This accounts for about one-fourth of the increase in health-care costs. The percent of the total population who are sixty-five or older only accounted for 12.4 percent of the population in 2000. By 2030, that will nearly double, to 20 percent of the population. As people age, they suffer more from the consequences of chronic diseases, and consequently need more health care.[11]

3. The number of malpractice lawsuits is rising. To avoid the cost of legal defense, doctors were more likely to over-test, even if they didn't really think the tests were needed. That meant they ordered MRIs, or Magnetic Resonance Imaging ($1,000 each), and colonoscopies ($1,500 each) rather than risk getting sued because they didn't order the test. It also meant medical offices were forced to spend more on malpractice insurance to protect themselves.

4. Doctors aren't paid for prescribing prevention. There wasn't as much financial reward for the preventive measures that have been shown to lower health-care costs. In other words, doctors didn't get paid for "prescribing" that patients eat healthier and exercise more. To keep their practices profitable and stay in business, there has been relentless pressure on doctors to rely on prescriptions and testing. For example, they were paid if they prescribed cholesterol-lowering medication when they told their patients to lose weight. This worked fine for many Americans who traditionally preferred their health-care solutions to come in a pill anyway.

5. Medical care is uncoordinated. One of the largest inefficiencies in the healthcare industry was the high administrative costs of health-care providers. Each doctor and specialist is affiliated with his or her own hospital and medical practice system, usually aligned with a specific area of expertise. For example, your doctor, who's affiliated with the local hospital because of its regional emergency room, might refer you to a pulmonologist who's affiliated with the hospital downtown that has lung research facilities. You assume they all coordinate care with each other, but they usually don't.

In another case, different specialists might order the exact same test for a patient if the first test was done in a lab they didn't use and trust. Other inefficiencies arose because most doctors didn't have electronic records. Haven't you wondered why most medical records were either mailed or faxed when the rest of the world used email? If records got lost, the test was often repeated. That's another reason some doctors found it was just easier to order new tests.

6. The health services payment system is out of whack. Traditionally, health care was the only industry where payment was made for each test, surgery, or prescription regardless of how well it worked or how good the outcome. This fee-for-service system meant doctors were financially rewarded for the number of procedures they prescribed instead of how effective these procedures actually were.

Who paid for these procedures? The US federal and state government paid the most, nearly 35 percent between Medicare (20 percent) and Medicaid (15 percent) combined. There was very little price shopping. A study of Medicare spending among states revealed some were much more expensive than others, but the outcomes were pretty much the same.

Health insurance companies, whether employer-based or privately bought, paid more than a third (33 percent) of medical bills.

That means only 12 percent of all medical services were paid for by the people who used them. Here, too, there was very little price comparison shopping. Unlike houses, automobile, or big-screen televisions, most people didn't really shop for the cheapest doctor or medical lab because they weren't directly billed for it. The true price was hidden from the buyers, who only paid a set fee (co-payment), and the insurance company paid the rest. Often the bill for the coinsurance didn't show up until long after the service was performed. Even doctors weren't sure of the prices for the tests and procedures they ordered. Can you think of anything else you buy where you don't know how much you paid? This gives medical providers very little incentive to lower costs.[12]

For these reasons, the CEA estimated that up to 30 percent of health-care costs could be saved without lowering the quality of care. It's no wonder that prices escalated out of control.[13]

7. Chronic illnesses are on the upswing. The most important reason for the high cost of health care, by far, is the epidemic of chronic diseases. Years ago, death arrived quickly from an outbreak of the flu, diphtheria, or an infection. Today, people are more likely to be slowly killed by the complications of chronic illnesses like heart disease, cancer, emphysema, stroke, Alzheimer's, and diabetes.

Nearly half of the US population has either asthma, heart disease, or diabetes. Those three diseases alone make up 85 percent of national health-care spending. Even more adults (60 percent) are either overweight or clinically obese, conditions that are highly correlated with chronic illnesses.[14]

Four of the Five Worst Killers Are Chronic Diseases

The five leading causes of death are heart disease, cancer, COPD, stroke, and accidents. These five alone caused 62 percent of all 2.6 million deaths in 2013 (most recent data available). Four of these five killers are caused by chronic diseases.[15]

You've heard about these diseases over and over. Blah, blah, blah, right? But do you really know exactly what they are, how they work, and how many people are affected? Do you really get how simple it is to reduce your likelihood of getting any of them, including cancer and Alzheimer's? If people knew and acted on the following information, then the leading cause of death would be accidents only. Let's start with the biggest killer.

Heart disease: It causes nearly one-fourth (611,105 people in 2013) of all deaths. The most common preventable conditions include:

- Coronary heart disease, where the arteries supplying blood to the heart get clogged and hardened with plaque buildup.
- Heart attacks, where plaque breaks off and blocks the flow of blood to the heart. If it's not cleared, it can kill heart tissue.

- Heart failure, where the heart muscle cannot pump blood the way it should.
- Heart disease and strokes. These cost $432 billion a year, but prevention is amazingly cost-effective. For example, reducing cholesterol levels by 10 percent lowers heart disease by 30 percent.[16]

Alzheimer's: There's growing evidence that heart disease also causes Alzheimer's disease. Nearly 80 percent of the nearly eighty-five thousand people who died of Alzheimer's in past years also had cardiovascular disease. Amazingly, the plaques and tangles of Alzheimer's, even if they're present in the brain during the autopsy, don't cause dementia *unless* the brain also shows evidence of vascular disease. As a result, many experts believe that reducing the incidence of heart disease may be the best way to prevent Alzheimer's dementia.

This makes sense. Your brain uses at least 20 percent of the blood from every heartbeat. That means 20 percent of all the food you eat and breaths you take go to support brain function. If this is cut off by heart disease, your brain is going to suffer.[17]

Alzheimer's affects more than five million seniors, as well as the eleven million family members who take care of them. In 2015, this added $226 billion in health-care costs to Medicare, Medicaid, insurance companies, and out-of-pocket costs to the families themselves. If you calculated the cost of the time spent by caregivers, it would add another $144 billion.

Of the total, $41 billion is spent by Medicaid, for the most part to pay for severe Alzheimer's patients in nursing homes. The disease is so devastating by this stage that families can no longer care for their loved ones. To qualify for Medicaid, seniors must first go through all their personal savings to reach the poverty level.

Half of all nursing home residents have Alzheimer's or other dementia, and half of those patients are on Medicaid. This will only worsen as more Baby Boomers age and contract the disease. By 2050, the number of seniors with Alzheimer's will nearly triple to 13.5 million, more than one out of ten. Half of them will have severe Alzheimer's, which means they have trouble having a conversation, eating without help, and even controlling their bodily functions.

By 2050, the costs will increase to a shocking $1.101 trillion, including $589 billion from Medicare. The costs to Medicaid for nursing home care for the most severe Alzheimer's patients will triple to $176 billion.[18]

Cancer: This disease kills almost as many people (22.5 percent of total 2013 mortality) as heart disease. In addition, roughly 1.7 million people are diagnosed with it each year.[19]

The medical cost of treating people with cancer was $88.7 billion in 2011 (most recent statistics available). In addition, the cost of lost productivity due to premature death was $130 billion. Here are the top five cancer killers, according to the American Cancer Society (ACS):

1. Lung cancer killed 159,000 people in 2014. It's almost entirely caused by smoking, according to the ACS. That's because there's an 87 percent correlation.[20]
2. Cancer of the genital system, including ovarian, prostate, and uterine cancer, killed fifty-nine thousand people in 2014. Risk factors include smoking, obesity, hormone replacement therapy, and family history.

Those with asthma, heart disease, and diabetes are responsible for nearly 85 percent of health-care costs.

---

3. Colorectal cancer kills fifty thousand people per year. Risk factors include age (90 percent of cases are found in people over fifty), obesity, alcoholism, and smoking. Processed food contributes to your chances of getting colorectal cancer, while fruits, vegetables, and dairy products reduce your chances.[21]
4. Breast cancer killed forty thousand people in 2014. This disease correlates with hormone replacement therapy, obesity, smoking, and genetic factors.
5. Pancreatic cancer killed nearly forty thousand people, and liver cancer killed twenty-three thousand in 2014. Risk factors include smoking (20 percent of pancreatic cancer), genetics, pancreatitis, diabetes, obesity, and alcoholism.

COPD (Chronic Obstructive Pulmonary Disease): This is responsible for nearly 150,000 deaths and costs $154 billion a year. COPD refers to either emphysema, chronic bronchitis, or both. Emphysema is damage to the walls between the lung's air sacs, which is where air is absorbed into the body. The damage makes it more difficult to absorb oxygen and exude carbon dioxide. Chronic bronchitis is inflammation of the airways, creating thick mucus.

COPD develops slowly, so you don't even know you have it until it's too late. By that point, you can't even walk, cook, or take care of yourself because you're always short of breath. That feeling of suffocation leads to panic attacks and trips to the emergency room for steroid injections and oxygen for temporary relief. There is no cure for COPD, and it is progressive.[22]

Smoking causes 90 percent of COPD deaths. The risk is increased if smokers started during childhood or teenage years. Nevertheless, 39 percent of the current fifteen million COPD sufferers keep smoking, even though they know it will make the disease progress faster.[23]

Nearly one out of five (17.4 percent) Americans are smokers. Although there's no disease called "smoking," it still kills 1,300 people a day. Smoking is so highly connected with the major chronic diseases that the CDC considers it *the* leading cause of preventable deaths in the United States.[24]

The correlations between smoking and many of the leading causes of death give insurance companies the legal right to charge you up to 50 percent higher premiums if you smoke. That's because this habit costs businesses an extra $6,000 per year per smoking employee, according to the *Tobacco Control Journal*. How? Taking smoke breaks cost $3,216 in lost productivity, $540 a year in absenteeism, and $480 a year in lowered productivity while actually working. The resultant health insurance costs are an extra $2,150 per smoker.[25]

Stroke: Nearly 800,000 Americans have strokes each year, costing $36.5 billion. Sadly, nearly 130,000 perish, contributing to 5 percent of all deaths. Most of these are ischemic strokes, which means blood flow to the brain is blocked. Nearly half (49 percent) of Americans have one of the risk factors for stroke: high blood pressure, high cholesterol, or smoking.

Accidents: Another 5 percent of deaths are caused by accidents, including injuries, falls, car accidents, or poisoning.

Diabetes: This disease is responsible for 2.9 percent of all deaths each year, and costs $174 billion annually. Even though it can be treated effectively, roughly two out of three diabetics still haven't gotten their blood sugar levels under control. If current trends continue, one out of every three babies born today will develop diabetes in their lifetime. Smoking contributes to type 2 diabetes.

Flu and Pneumonia: Combined, these two diseases cause nearly fifty-seven thousand deaths each year. Those at high risk are people with asthma or COPD; those with heart disease, diabetes, or kidney disease; the morbidly obese; and those with weakened immune systems, such as cancer survivors.[26]

Kidney disease: Failing kidneys cause a little more than forty-seven thousand deaths each year. The CDC estimates that 10 percent of the population has kidney disease, but many don't know it because the symptoms don't show until it's too late. The best way to find out is through blood tests during your annual physical. The two main risk factors are diabetes and high blood pressure. The risk for kidney disease is two to three times higher for diabetics who smoke than for those who don't.[27]

Obesity: This condition is highly correlated to the major chronic diseases. Imagine the outcry if the government tried to eliminate obesity. In fact, many overweight people proclaim they have a right to their body size.

However, this right comes at a very high cost to them and to society. Fatty tissue is where the body stores excess toxins and hormones. That's one way obesity contributes to three of the five big killers: heart disease, stroke, and some types of cancer (breast, colon, kidney, and endometrial). Obesity is also a risk factor for diabetes, liver disease, and osteoarthritis. As a result, obesity adds $147 billion to health-care costs annually.[28]

Nearly eighty million adults are obese, which is defined as a Body Mass Index (BMI) of thirty or more. For example, an average-height woman (5'5") who weighs more than 180 pounds or an average-height man (5'10") who weighs more than 205 pounds would be considered obese. One in twenty adults are extremely obese, with a BMI that's higher than forty. That's 240 pounds for an average-height woman, or 270 pounds for an average-height man.

In fact, people who are of normal or below-normal weight are in the minority in America. That's because two in three adults are overweight (although not yet obese), with a BMI between 25.0 and 29.9. That's an average-height woman who weighs from 150 to 180 or an average-height man who weighs from 175 to 205.

Nearly thirteen million children and adolescents are obese, which is defined as a BMI at or above the ninety-fifth percentile.

Obesity is getting worse. The rate in adults has doubled, while the rate in children has tripled in the last twenty years. That's why the CDC considers obesity an epidemic. In 2013, the AMA classified it as a disease.[29]

Cost of Managing Chronic Diseases

Chronic diseases are a major reason for the rising cost of health care, even before they cause deaths. In fact, they are responsible for three out of every four dollars spent on health care. That's because 49 percent of all Americans suffer from at least one chronic disease. This adds up to an extra $7,900 in health-care costs for each of them. That's five times more than someone without a chronic disease.

One big reason for high costs is that these diseases limit mobility and earning power. Nearly 25 percent of chronic disease patients can't go to school or work, and might even need help with dressing or bathing.

The impact of these chronic diseases was reported by Eileen Crimmins at the University of Southern California. She compared the physical limitations of men who were at least eighty years old in 1998 to those in the same age bracket in 2006. In 1998, only 28 percent of the men had these limitations, but by 2006 she found limitations existed in 42 percent of the later group. In other words, despite ten years of improvements in medicine, the elderly were less able to get around than before. Research done by the Harvard School of Public Health found that the same thing happened with mental health—the elderly suffered more from depression and dementia, probably due to the loss of mobility.[30]

Another reason costs are so high is that many sufferers simply ignore their symptoms until they wind up in the emergency room. That's because they are overwhelmed with how complicated and expensive the conditions are to both treat and manage.

For example, many patients get tired of taking so many medications, or they simply can't afford it. When they cut back, they put themselves at risk for heart attacks, strokes, or comas that send them to the emergency room.

Impact of High Medical Costs: The Number One Cause of Bankruptcy

A 2012 survey found that more than one out of four people were in families burdened by medical bills. Most of them were paying the bills as they could over time. However, 16.5 percent were in families who had problems paying those bills in the past year, and 8.9 percent just couldn't pay them at all.[31]

Harvard University researchers were shocked to find that medical costs caused 62 percent of all personal bankruptcies in 2007. Even more disturbing was that 78 percent of those who went bankrupt *had* health insurance—it just failed to cover all their bills. Not surprising was that 60 percent of those with insurance were let down by private or employer-sponsored insurance, not Medicare or Medicaid. In other words, the government did a better job of protecting those it insured than did private insurance companies.

As a result, the families who were let down, and went bankrupt, were not the poor who are usually well-covered by Medicaid. Instead, two-thirds were homeowners and three-fifths were college graduates.

They were middle-class Americans who got hit with massive, and unexpected, out-of-pocket medical expenses. The cost to those with private insurance averaged nearly $17,800 per family, while those who lost insurance during the process faced bills as high as $22,650 each. Naturally, those without insurance were hit with the highest bills, averaging $26,970 per family.

How did those with insurance wind up with so many bills? After high deductibles, coinsurance payments, and annual or lifetime limits, the insurance ran out. Other companies denied claims, or canceled the insurance.

A frightening 90 percent of those with homes had to take out a second mortgage. Nearly 30 percent maxed out their credit cards, while 8 percent were forced into bankruptcy because the illness cost them their jobs.

The most expensive diseases were diabetes, averaging nearly $27,000 per family, and neurological disorders like multiple sclerosis, which cost almost $34,200 on average. The biggest expense was hospitalization, which caused half of the bankruptcies.[32]

America's Health Care: The Most Expensive, But Not the Best, in the World

Did you ever notice that the doctor, when you finally got into see him or her, usually seemed rushed and often spent no more than fifteen minutes with you? That's because they were paid, whether it was by insurance companies or Medicare, based on how many appointments they logged and how many procedures and prescriptions they wrote. Many were under pressure from their business managers to book a certain number of patients a day, and their pay was docked if they didn't meet the target.

As a result, the quality of care suffered. A 1999 study by the Institute of Medicine revealed that forty-four thousand to ninety-eight thousand deaths per year were caused by "never events," medical errors that should never have happened, because they were absolutely preventable if prescribed safety standards had been used.

The largest of these errors included performing surgery on the wrong organ or even the wrong patient, prescribing the wrong drug or dosage, and transmitting hospital-acquired infections such as MRSA *(Methicillin-resistant Staphylococcus aureus)*, an antibiotic-resistant infection. They occurred because doctors were too rushed to perform common safety procedures, such as washing hands between patients, counting the number of surgical instruments before and after the procedure to make sure none were left inside the patient, and double-checking drugs before they were administered.[33]

If quality of care wasn't great for most, it was virtually nonexistent for those without insurance. That's because without insurance, or a means to pay for medical care, people simply didn't go to the doctor. As a result, each year more than 100,000 of these uninsured Americans died simply because they couldn't afford the care that would have saved their lives.

Even those who were insured often were left without care when they needed it. They didn't even realize their insurance wouldn't cover a procedure until they sent in a claim. Others received great care until they hit their annual or lifetime limit. More on that in chapter 5.

The high cost of health care is eating up the federal budget, destroying America's small businesses, and sentencing many to an early death. Therefore, the number-one goal of Obamacare is to drive those costs down. Fortunately, the best way to do that also improves the quality of care. That's why you are going to benefit from Obamacare, even if you do nothing. Don't worry, though—this book also give you the steps you need to make sure you get everything you can from the Affordable Care Act.

Chapter 2: References

1. "Table S-3. Discretionary Funding by Major Agency. Table S-8. Budget Summary by Category. Summary Tables, The Budget for Fiscal Year 2009," Office of Management and Budget. http://useconomy.about.com/library/FY_2009_Budget.pdf, accessed September 3, 2014.

2. Kimberly Amadeo, FY 2015 Budget, US Economy.About.com. http://useconomy.about.com/od/usfederalbudget/fl/Federal-Budget-FY-2015.htm, accessed February 2, 2015.

3. "Table S-5. Proposed Budget by Category, FY 2016 Budget," Office of Management and Budget. https://www.whitehouse.gov/sites/default/files/omb/budget/fy2016/assets/tables.pdf, accessed February 2, 2015.

4. "The Facts on Medicare Spending," Kaiser Family Foundation, July 28, 2014. http://kff.org/medicare/fact-sheet/medicare-spending-and-financing-fact-sheet/, accessed September 2, 2014. Damian Paletta, "Falling Costs Boost Medicare Outlook," *Wall Street Journal,* July 29, 2014.

5. "Exhibit 5. The Facts on Medicare Spending," Kaiser.

6. "Exhibit 2. The Facts on Medicare Spending," Kaiser.

7. Karen Politz and Cynthia Cox, "Medical Debt Among People With Health Insurance," Kaiser Family Foundation, January 7, 2014. http://kff.org/private-insurance/report/medical-debt-among-people-with-health-insurance, accessed September 3, 2014.

8. "National Health Expenditures," CMS.gov. http://www.cms.gov/Research-Statistics-Data-and-Systems/Statistics-Trends-and-Reports/NationalHealthExpendData/Downloads/tables.pdf, accessed September 3, 2014.

9. Ezekiel Emanuel, "Why I Hope to Die at 75," *The Atlantic*, September 17, 2014. http://www.theatlantic.com/features/archive/2014/09/why-i-hope-to-die-at-75/379329/ accessed October 11, 2014.

10. Julie Appleby, "Seven Factors Driving Up Your Health Care Costs," Kaiser Health News, October 24, 2012. http://www.kaiserhealthnews.org/stories/2012/october/25/health-care-costs.aspx, accessed October 6, 2014.

11. Carrie A. Werner, "The Older Population: 2010," US Census, November 2011. https://www.census.gov/prod/cen2010/briefs/c2010br-09.pdf, accessed October 6, 2014. Jennifer M. Ortman, Victoria A. Velkoff, and Howard Hogan, "An Aging Nation: The

Older Population in the United States," US Census, May 2014. https://www.census.gov/prod/2014pubs/p25-1140.pdf, accessed October 6, 2014.

12. "National Health Expenditures 2013 Highlights," CMS.gov. http://www.cms.gov/Research-Statistics-Data-and-Systems/Statistics-Trends-and-Reports/NationalHealthExpendData/Downloads/highlights.pdf, accessed June 16, 2015.

13. "The Economic Case for Health Care Reform," Council of Economic Advisers. https://www.whitehouse.gov/administration/eop/cea/TheEconomicCaseforHealthCareReform/, accessed June 16, 2015.

14. "Chronic Disease Overview," CDC.gov, 2013. http://www.cdc.gov/chronicdisease/overview/index.htm, accessed July 6, 2015.

15 "Deaths and Mortality," CDC.gov, 2013. http://www.cdc.gov/nchs/fastats/deaths.htm, accessed June 16, 2015.

16. "Eight Heart Conditions That Kill You," *Muscle Mag Fitness*, December 4, 2014. http://www.musclemagfitness.com/disease-and-conditions/heart-disease/eight-heart-conditions-that-can-kill-you.html, accessed December 4, 2014. "The Effects of Heart Disease," For a Healthier America. http://www.forahealthieramerica.com/ds/paying-price-of-heart-disease.html, accessed November 4, 2014.

17. "Prevention and Risk of Alzheimer's and Dementia," ALZ.org. http://www.alz.org/research/science/alzheimers_prevention_and_risk.asp, accessed November 4, 2014.

18. "Changing the Trajectory of Alzheimer's Disease: A National Imperative," Alzheimer's Association, 2010. http://www.alz.org/documents_custom/trajectory.pdf, accessed November 4, 2014.

19. "Cancer Facts and Figures 2014," American Cancer Society, 2014. http://www.cancer.org/acs/groups/content/@research/documents/webcontent/acspc-042151.pdf, accessed July 29, 2014.

20. Lynne Eldrige, MD, "Smoking and Lung Cancer," Lungcancer.about.com. http://lungcancer.about.com/od/causesoflungcance1/a/smokinglungcancer.htm, accessed December 4, 2014.

21. Harris Meyer, "Under Health Law, Colonoscopies Are Free," Kaiser Health News, April 25, 2011. http://kaiserhealthnews.org/news/health-law-colonoscopy/, accessed November 4, 2014.

22. "What Is COPD?" National Heart, Lung and Blood Institute. http://www.nhlbi.nih.gov/health/health-topics/topics/copd, accessed July 29, 2014.

23. "Smoking and COPD," Centers for Disease Control and Prevention. http://www.cdc .gov/tobacco/campaign/tips/diseases/copd.html, accessed July 29, 2014.

24. Centers for Disease Control and Prevention, "Smoking-Attributable Mortality, Years of Potential Life Lost, and Productivity Losses—United States, 2000–2004," *Morbidity and Mortality Weekly Report,* 57 (45): 1226-8, 2008.

25. Rachel Wells, "Smokers Cost Employers $6,000 a Year Each," *Sydney Morning Herald*, June 17, 2013. http://www.smh.com.au/national/smokers-cost-employers-3000 -a-year-each-20130617-2od7l.html, accessed July 29, 2014.

26. "People at High Risk of Developing Flu-Related Complications," Centers for Disease Control and Prevention. http://www.cdc.gov/flu/about/disease/high_risk.htm, accessed July 29, 2014.

27. "National Chronic Kidney Disease Fact Sheet 2014," Centers for Disease Control and Prevention. http://www.cdc.gov/diabetes/pubs/pdf/kidney_factsheet.pdf, July 29, 2014. "Leading Causes of Death," Centers for Disease Control and Prevention, 2010, Latest data available. http://www.cdc.gov/nchs/data/dvs/LCWK9_2011.pdf, accessed August 19, 2014.

28. "Obesity: Halting the Epidemic by Making Health Easier," Centers for Disease Control and Prevention. http://www.cdc.gov/nccdphp/publications/AAG/pdf/obesity.pdf, accessed December 6, 2014. "Overweight and Obesity Statistics," National Institute of Diabetes and Digestive and Kidney Diseases. http://www.niddk.nih.gov/health-information/health-statistics/Pages/overweight-obesity-statistics.aspx, accessed June 16, 2015.

29. "Adult Obesity Facts," Centers for Disease Control and Prevention. http://www.cdc .gov/obesity/adult/index.html, accessed July 29, 2014; "Obesity Is Now Considered a Disease," Cleveland Clinic, June 25, 2013. http://health.clevelandclinic.org/2013/06/ obesity-is-now-considered-a-disease/, accessed May 25, 2015.

30. Ezekiel Emanuel, "Why I Hope to Die at 75," *The Atlantic*.

31. Robin A. Cohen Ph.D. and Shitney K. Kirzinger, MPH, "Financial Burden of Medical Care: A Family Perspective," *NCHS Date Brief*, No. 142, January 2014. http://www .cdc.gov/nchs/data/databriefs/db142.pdf, accessed October 6, 2014.

32. Catherine Arnst, "Study Links Medical Costs and Personal Bankruptcy," *Bloomberg BusinessWeek*, June 4, 2009. http://www.businessweek.com/bwdaily/dnflash/content /jun2009/db2009064_666715.htm, accessed October 6, 2014.

33. Trish Torrey, "Issues in Patient Safety—Serious Reportable, Adverse or Never Events," About.com, December 16, 2013. http://patients.about.com/od/empowermentbasics/a/patientsafety.htm, accessed October 6, 2014.

Chapter 3

THREE WAYS THE ACA MODERNIZES HEALTH CARE AND LOWERS COSTS

On February 9, 2007, Lisa Galison's gynecologist found a suspicious lump in her breast during her annual exam. He ordered her to get a mammogram the following week. Filled with fear, Lisa took time off from work to find a center, make an appointment, and go get the mammogram. Based on the findings, the doctor ordered a biopsy. Lisa took more time off from work and went to a different facility downtown to have the minor surgery done. The biopsy went to another facility to be read by the pathologist.

Unfortunately, he found cancer. Lisa went to a fifth doctor, the breast surgeon, for a lumpectomy. A sixth doctor, an oncologist, administered the chemotherapy. A seventh professional, the radiation oncologist, administered radiation therapy over the next six weeks.

At each visit, Lisa provided the surgical and pathology reports, x-rays, CT scans, lab results, and her medical history. Several times, one of the doctors ordered his own scans from an office he trusted more.

During this whole ordeal, Lisa dealt with the scary thought of having breast cancer and what it meant to her, her family, and her life. On top of that, she also had to suddenly become a health-care coordinator for herself. She scheduled the visits and then tried to understand the test results and what the diagnoses meant for her. She also had to find some counseling to help her deal emotionally with this devastating life-threatening condition.[1]

Fortunately, Lisa's procedure was a success, and she's been cancer-free for five years. Unfortunately, the ordeal of dealing with the insurance companies also lasted nearly that long. Her insurance company didn't agree with her doctors' ordering of separate tests, and didn't pay for some of them. On top of losing money from taking so much time off from work, Lisa paid $1,700 in medical bills that weren't covered by insurance. No wonder medical bills are the number one reason for bankruptcy in America.

This is what fragmented care looks like.

The ACA makes it possible for hospitals, doctors, and pharmacists to work together to get you better faster. It makes sure all records are put on computers so they can be transferred electronically. This means you will have one record that allows all of your doctors to share their diagnoses and treatments. Your clerical and payment information will also be part of this record. In addition, the ACA pays hospitals based on how well you get, instead of how many tests and procedures you get.

The health-care industry recognizes that integrated care is the way of the future. The best of the best already foresee that the industry must evolve from a system where every doctor must try to be an expert in every health condition. It's become way too complex for that.

Medical teams will be able to take advantage of knowledge from sophisticated data analysis. This is already being done in most other industries, and explains the success of successful companies from Disney to Target.

For example, Disney collects data from visitors to its Magic Kingdom with wristbands that tell the park managers what rides are popular, what food is being ordered, and what's being purchased. This allows them to immediately add staff where needed and to determine over time which rides are profitable. They also know what types of customers will go to the website later to purchase things, and whether these customers stay in a Disney-related hotel. [2]

Before Obamacare, the medical profession didn't even have data about patients to transfer electronically among team members. That made it more difficult to work in an integrated approach, since team members couldn't easily share information about patients.

Big data will allow health-care companies to determine where specialists are needed, how effective they are, and what services should be added or eliminated. Companies like Disney have known for a long time that it's a great way to provide better service while cutting costs.

As health care grew more complex, many doctors moved away from their own private practices, which were becoming unaffordable and too risky for them. Most doctors are great at what they've been trained to do, which is to diagnose diseases and recommend treatment. But today's economy also requires them to be excellent marketers, efficiency experts, and personnel managers.

As a result, more and more doctors signed up to be wage-based employees of a major hospital. They let the hospital handle the administration, so they could focus on patient care.

However, even hospitals must change. Harvard professor and expert in competitive advantage Michael Porter recommends that hospitals focus on a specialty. Today's health care is too complicated for each and every hospital to be excellent in all areas of care. This is especially true for small, rural hospitals that don't have enough customers to fund full care.

Instead, they must form networks with each other. The small community hospitals can continue to treat broken bones, appendicitis attacks, and pregnancies. They can stabilize heart attacks, strokes, and other serious emergency situations. At that point, they can send these patients to an affiliated hospital that specializes in cardiac care, neurology, or complex treatment plans.[3]

When most people think of Obamacare, they think of the health-care exchanges and the controversy surrounding them. However, if you talk to anyone in the health-care industry itself, you'll soon learn that the biggest impact of the ACA is on doctors and hospitals. In the next three sections, you'll learn exactly what the ACA is doing to bring health-care into the twenty-first century.

Understand Integrated Care

Sam Thompson called his daughter in a panic. He felt as if he couldn't breathe, so she rushed him to the Trinity Regional Hospital emergency room in Ft. Dodge, Iowa. That's when he found out he had congestive heart failure. The next day, his doctor sent him home with a list of things to do and a stack of prescriptions.

Tammy Bennett, a Care Coordinator Case Manager for Trinity Pioneer ACO, called Sam right away to set up an appointment to visit him the next day. During the visit, she went over Sam's discharge instructions to make sure he understood and would follow them.

She reviewed his medications with him. She explained congestive heart failure to him, so he understood how his life had changed. Tammy's caring and expertise allowed Sam to trust her.

Tammy also made sure his home was safe, guiding him to remove rugs that could cause him to slip and fall. She also checked that he had support besides his daughter. She helped him set up appointments with community health centers, so he would receive the continuing care he needed to manage his chronic condition. She called him once a week for at least the next four weeks, just to make sure he was OK.

Integrated care means outreach to the most vulnerable patients. Hospital-paid case coordinators are the outreach arm of integrated care. They help patients make a list of who to call to get transportation, and they explain the disease and the patient's care requirements to the family.

Research shows that, without this attention, patients will end up back in the hospital within five days on average. That's because during their discharge they are given so much information in such a short time that it's difficult to understand everything about their condition and what they must do to recover. Although the goal of integrated care is lower health-care costs, the result is better treatment for the patients.[4]

Integrated Care Helps Family Caregivers

Maggie Peterson's seventy-eight-year-old mother fell and broke her neck. Although Maggie has four other siblings, she was the only one who lived in the same town and wasn't married or had children.

Although her mother wanted her to move in with her, Maggie had a full-time job that she couldn't just quit. Since her mother lived an hour away, Maggie couldn't even drive over every day. However, trying to find care for her mother was a full-time job in itself. Her mother was only in the hospital long enough to be fitted with a brace. Upon discharge, she needed constant care to help her with eating, bathing, and getting dressed. Finding immediate care was nearly impossible until her mother called a friend who agreed to take over when Maggie left for work on Monday.

Fortunately, Maggie's mom had long-term care insurance, and they quickly set up round-the-clock nursing care. Most people aren't this fortunate.

A 2009 survey by the Association for the Advancement of Retired People (AARP) found that more than forty-two million Americans provide day-to-day care for their parents. Nearly sixty-two million provide some care during the year.

Ninety percent of ailing seniors want to stay at home. Similarly, most children don't want their parents to go to an institution. However, no matter how well-intentioned they are, caregivers burn out fast. Among female caregivers fifty and over, 20 percent reported depression.

Caregiving also costs adult children financially. According to a 2007 Evercare report, those who lived with their elderly parents spent $5,885 a year on caregiving costs. Those who lived nearby spent $4,570, while those who were long-distance spent the most—$8,728 annually.[5]

Nursing homes aren't even an option for many of those without long-term care insurance. These skilled facilities cost $72,000 a year on average, and most people mistakenly believe they're covered by Medicare. Mostly they aren't. Medicare only covers this type of nursing care when it's medically necessary. That means changing bandages or other medical procedures that require a skilled nurse. It usually only occurs following a hospital stay or surgery.

Most people in nursing homes only require custodial care, like help with bathing and dressing. That's not covered by Medicare or most health insurance.

Assisted-living facilities help seniors that aren't bedridden but need help with two or more activities of daily living, such as eating, bathing, and dressing. While less expensive, they still cost $38,000 a year. Home health care is more reasonable, at $30,000 a year according to LifePlans, but not by much.

These services are out of the reach of most seniors without long-term care insurance. In 2010, half of those sixty-five and older lived on incomes of less than $22,000 a year. Similarly, half had less than $53,000 in retirement savings, according to the Kaiser Family Foundation.

However, regardless of whether they planned for it or not, and regardless of whether they have children who are willing and able to care for them or not, the fact remains—more than ten million Americans need long-term care.

What happens to those who have no one to care for them? First, they quickly spend their life savings to pay for care, whether in a facility or at home. When this runs out, they may have to sell their house and every other asset they own. Only then are they eligible for Medicaid's coverage of an approved facility.

Who pays for it? The federal government (that means taxpayers) through Medicaid. As a result, the federal government picks up the tab for 40 percent of all long-term nursing home care. Forty-five states allow Medicaid to pay for some form of assisted living since it's about half the cost, and it helps keep many seniors out of nursing homes.[6]

Fortunately, the ACA expanded Medicaid to cover those who make 138 percent or less of the federal poverty level. This helps more seniors afford medical costs, so they can use other income to pay for non-medical needs, allowing them to stay at home. Expanded Medicaid allows more seniors to get assisted living in the thirty states, plus the District of Columbia, that adopted the ACA's expanded Medicaid coverage.

However, that's not to say the ACA allows Medicaid to pay for all assisted living. The states vary widely in what they allow Medicaid to cover. Most states use Medicaid waivers for assisted living, and they cap the number of waivers they grant. Therefore, there's often a long waiting list.

States are not uniform in what they cover. They could cover anything from residential care, to adult foster care, to personal care services. Some states only allow Medicaid to pay for personal care received in assisted living facilities, while others include nursing services.

States are not allowed to pay room and board costs, but they can cap the costs charged by assisted living facilities. As a result, a lot of assisted-living centers won't accept Medicaid. Those that do may obviously be limited in what they can provide. Therefore, it's best to plan to pay for assisted living costs yourself if there's any way possible—or get long-term care insurance.

For example, California pays for assisted living through Medi-Cal via an Assisted Living Waiver. The waiver can only be used if the patient qualifies for nursing home care, but it would cost less to either be in an assisted living facility or at home. However, the waiver is only available in seven major counties because there aren't facilities in every county. Therefore, the patient must be willing to move to a facility in a county where it is available. In addition, the patient must contribute around $1,000 a month to room and board costs.

Rhode Island uses Medicaid funds for nursing-home care only. It has its own program called SSI Enhanced Assisted Living Program that contributes $1,200 a month for assisted living. Like California, the state also provides a Medicaid waiver. Since every state is so different, you'd need to research exactly what your state covers. A good resource is a website called Paying for Senior Care.[7]

What's the Best Way to Provide Integrated Care?

The ACA created the Center for Medicare and Medicaid Innovation to test the best ways to deliver integrated care. The goal of integrated care is to improve quality while reducing the rate of growth in Medicare spending.

Anthem and other health-care providers are taking seriously the challenge of providing integrated care. An Anthem survey found that 40 percent of patients support the idea of integrated care. It makes their lives easier by providing all their doctors with the details of their medical history. Most people can't remember all their vaccinations, medications, and diagnoses and find it difficult to update their different doctors and specialists on all these details.

Anthem offers vision and primary care benefits. It then makes electronic claims data available to doctors, who can view all the information about their patients, and even attach it to their own medical records.[8]

Accountable Care Organizations: Radically Changing Health Care

The advancement of accountable care organizations (ACO) is the biggest change being made by Obamacare, and yet you probably had no idea it was happening. If it works, it will improve your care, lower your premiums, and reduce the federal budget deficit.

Thanks to the Affordable Care Act, more than 360 ACOs have been established since 2010. They are working in a large-scale pilot program with Medicare that serves 5.3 million senior citizens. These include physician-led organizations, community health centers, and hospitals.

Medicare's pilot program is already working to lower costs. The growth in Medicare spending per beneficiary hit historic lows from 2010 to 2013. It's expected that the growth in spending will match the growth rate of the economy. This breaks a decades-long trend of Medicare spending growing much faster than the economy.

The coordinated care approach used by ACOs has been pioneered by leading hospitals and health-care organizations such as Kaiser Permanente. These healthcare organizations found that using ACOs results in fewer emergency room visits, readmissions, and hospital-acquired conditions. The ACA and Medicare are pushing it to a broader population. Health insurance companies are already noticing the model's success, recognizing it as the way of the future.

What Exactly Is an ACO?

An ACO is a group of health-care providers that agree to be held accountable for the health of their patient population. Medicare changes the payment method from the traditional fee-for-service to a payment system that rewards quality of care.

The bundled payment system pays a set fee for each episode of care, such as a heart attack, stroke, or knee replacement. The population-based payment system pays a set fee for each patient. If the ACO can treat patients for less than the set fee, it pockets the difference. This provides a strong incentive for the ACO to keep its patients healthy by coordinating care, focusing on prevention, and eliminating unnecessary tests and procedures.

ACOs must also implement electronic health records. This makes all medical history and Medicare data available to all of the patient's doctors via a shared database. That makes coordinated care much easier. Other benefits from electronic health records are discussed in more detail later in this chapter.

To make sure the ACO retains a high quality of care, Medicare requires it to meet certain quantifiable standards, such as the number of hospital readmissions, the number of hospital-acquired diseases, and scores on patient questionnaires. If the ACO falls below the standards set by Medicare, its payment is cut.

ACOs are not the same as a Medicare Advantage plan. ACOs are groups of hospitals and doctors that provide services covered by Original Medicare, such as hospitalization. Medicare Advantage plans are insurance plans that include Original Medicare but also provide coverage for benefits such as outpatient doctor visits, vision care, and prescriptions. The ACOs are paid by the Original Medicare program, follow those rules, and provide the services covered by Original Medicare.

It's important to understand the difference, because the hospital affiliated with your Medicare Advantage plan may decide to enter the ACO test model. If that happens, you'll notice many improvements from coordinated care, electronic records, and quieter hospital stays. However, this won't increase your insurance premiums.

How Do ACOs Work?

Usually a hospital leads the charge. It assembles a team of doctors, specialists, labs, and pharmacists to coordinate care within the formal legal structure of an ACO. The new ACO agrees to be accountable to Medicare for the quality, cost, and overall care of beneficiaries. It ensures that members stay healthy and avoid unnecessary hospital admissions. Medicare shares any cost savings with the ACO.

All providers share an integrated electronic health record system. That means everyone who cares for you will know your medical history, so you won't have to fill out endless forms that just ask for the same thing over and over again. You won't have to bring a list of your prescriptions with you. And you won't have to worry that a specialist or hospital doctor will recommend a procedure that works against the treatment plan you're already on.

Behind the scenes, Centers for Medicare and Medicaid Services (CMS) analysts review the data to come up with better ways to take care of you. For example, the data shows which procedures best reduce the spread of infections between patients in hospitals. The CMS publishes these evidence-based guidelines to ACOs. The guidelines are accessible to everyone within the ACO. That means doctors have additional resources based on real-life experiences to guide them in diagnosing and treating your disease.

Your doctors will inform you if they join an ACO, so you can opt out if you prefer. For example, some people are nervous about having their medical records shared with the data analysts. However, your medical information is protected by the Health Insurance Portability and Accountability Act (HIPAA) as it's always been. Only people who are actively involved with your treatment will see your personal records. The data analysts don't see your personal information, such as name, address, Social Security number, or phone number. [9]

Three ACO Pilot Programs

CMS evaluates many types of ACOs to find out what works best. It also adapts programs to meet the needs of different health-care systems, which vary by size, sophistication, and type of community served. Below are descriptions of three programs that give you an idea of how the ACA is providing a new approach to health-care delivery in America.

Medicare Shared Savings Program: This is the basic program established by section 3022 of the ACA. It's designed to help traditional fee-for-service providers transition to become ACOs. The providers sign a three-year contract with CMS where they agree to coordinate services for their Medicare patients. Success is gauged by thirty quality measures within four areas: patient experience, patient safety, preventive health, and at-risk populations. ACOs that meet their quality targets while reducing growth in expenses will have the most savings to share.

CMS estimates what it would cost to serve the ACO's Medicare population for the next three years. The estimate is based on past actual costs, which CMS has in its database. It projects increases in future costs based on national data trends. Since the estimates are based on the traditional fee-for-service basis, the ACO gets a good idea of what its costs would be if it hadn't entered the Shared Savings Program.

If the ACO's actual costs are from 2 percent to 3.9 percent lower than the CMS estimate, Medicare and the ACO split the savings 50/50. If its costs are higher, it still receives the estimate.

Once this is successful, the ACO can elect to step up to a shared risk program. In that case, it receives 60 percent of the savings. However, if its actual costs are higher than the benchmark, it must pay Medicare a portion of those overages.[10]

As of January 1, 2015, there were 404 Shared Savings Program ACOs in 49 states (except Hawaii) serving 7.3 million patients. The ten regional centers with the most ACOs were: Atlanta (109), Chicago (88), New York (60), Philadelphia (59), Dallas (54), San Francisco (49), Boston (37), Kansas City (31), Denver (12), and Seattle (7).[11]

Advance Payment ACO: Doctor-owned and rural providers that sign up for the Shared Savings Program can receive advance payments to help them get the technology and staff they need to become ACOs. They pay back the advance from their resultant savings. This allows the smaller providers to grow and become sophisticated enough to fully join the Shared Savings Program.

There are 35 ACOs in this pilot. Nine are in Florida; four in Texas; three each in Maryland and Kentucky; two each in Tennessee, California, and Connecticut; and one each in Arkansas, Indiana, Maine, Missouri, Mississippi, North Carolina, Nebraska, New Hampshire, Ohio, and Rhode Island.[12]

Pioneer ACO: This model is for organizations that already provide some level of integrated service. If proven to be successful, it is the wave of the future for health care in America.

Here's how it works. The ACO itself, as the legal representative entity, signs a three-year contract with CMS. For the first two years, payments are made on the Shared Savings model. In the third year, half of the payment from Medicare is population-based, while the other half remains fee-for-service.

Population-based payment means the hospital receives a payment for each patient in their assigned population. CMS determines who is in the ACO's population based on the prior three years of data. The ACO knows in advance who will be counted as part of its population base.

Patients are free to use doctors outside of the ACO. As long as the claims are submitted to Medicare, the ACO doctors will still have access to the information. This helps them to be more aware of all the conditions and care their patients are receiving. That's because all patient data is shared between Medicare and the ACO. Any doctor or specialist can use the electronic medical records to look up the history of a patient's medical conditions, prescriptions, and doctor visits.

The purpose of population-based payment is to make the ACO more responsible for the overall health of their patients. The healthier the patient, the lower the cost to the ACO, and the more profit it makes. This gives a powerful economic incentive for the ACO to coordinate care, focus on prevention, and teach patients how to be responsible for their own health.

Patients in ACOs receive greater protection. They are surveyed each year about the care they receive. CMS investigates ACOs that have too many complaints. CMS routinely analyzes the data to compare how well patients use the ACO compared to other similar healthcare providers. Patients can call Medicare directly if they are concerned or unhappy with their ACO. [13]

There were 160 health-care providers that expressed interest in being considered for the pilot. Of those, eighty actually submitted applications, and thirty-two were approved. As of 2015, nineteen were still in the program. Five were in Massachusetts, including Beth Israel Deaconess in Boston; three were in California, including Monarch Healthcare in Orange County and Brown and Toland in San Francisco; and three were in Minnesota, including Park Nicollet in Minneapolis. Eight other states had one each: Arizona, Iowa, Illinois, Maine, Michigan, New Hampshire, New York, and Wisconsin. [14]

By May 2015, the Pioneer ACO programs had saved Medicare $384 million, or $300 per patient. Doctors prescribed fewer unnecessary tests and procedures, and patients didn't need to return to the hospital as often after discharge.

Pioneer ACO programs also improved quality of care. Patients reported that doctors communicated with them better and were able to schedule appointments with them sooner than expected. Better guidance meant the patients were more likely to comply with instructions and complete all their follow-up care. [15]

Benefits of ACOs

There are many benefits for patients. Those with multiple doctors and specialists no longer feel like "the left hand doesn't know what the right hand is doing." They don't have to fill out the same information on a different form for every doctor they go to. They don't have to remember to send tests and results from their specialists to the doctors, and vice versa. The doctor that treats them at the emergency room or hospital has the same information as their primary care physician, and vice versa.

That means patients don't have to undergo the same test for different doctors. They don't worry about being prescribed medications or procedures that work against those prescribed by other doctors. They have additional help in coordinating their care, especially after a hospital stay or if they have a chronic disease. Patients can keep all their doctors—since the ACO allows them to go outside of the organization for care (unlike an HMO).

The primary benefit for the federal government is lower Medicare costs. The Congressional Budget Office (CBO) estimates that it will save as much as $5 billion in its first eight years. However, it expects most of those savings to occur in the later years as the program attracts more and more medical providers. The Pioneer and Shared Savings ACO models combined saved $417 million. Although this seems below target, it's still early, and savings should improve over time if the CBO's assumptions are accurate. [16]

Many health-care providers who were sitting on the fence now realize this is the way of the future. Many health insurers are adopting ACO-type contracts with their physician networks. For example, UnitedHealth Group, Aetna, and Anthem are working with oncologists to manage and coordinate care for cancer patients who are members of their plans.[17]

The ACA's focus on quality of care means hospitals must focus on it too. That's not to say they didn't before. It does mean that hospitals put in place new procedures to make sure they absolutely comply with the government's standards. For example, some have replaced all the squeaky wheels on food carts because patient complaints about noise are measured by the government. What might seem like a small thing becomes a big one if it results in lower reimbursement from Medicare.[18]

Problems with ACOs

The main complaint about ACOs is that the federal programs are just too complex, there are too many quality metrics, and the incentives are not great enough.

Some doctors point out that transitioning to ACOs creates more headaches for them. They also don't benefit that much from the shared savings. Instead, most of the savings go to the hospitals and health-care administration companies that skim the profits off the top to manage the ACOs.

The other concern is that the emphasis on ACOs creates health-care monopolies. It gives large organizations a competitive advantage, driving smaller practices out of business. Over time, as with any monopoly, this will drive up costs in an area.

Pioneer Program: Of the thirty-two providers who signed up for the Pioneer pilot in 2012, thirteen dropped out in the first three years. Most of them signed up for the Shared Savings program instead.

What went wrong? Despite following the guidelines, they were not able to lower Medicare spending enough to meet the national benchmark. Others found their costs were higher than the benchmark. However, most did improve in their quality measures, such as screening for tobacco use and controlling high blood pressure.

The Pioneer program saved $96 million in its first year, but only $68 million of that was shared back with the ACOs. That's because only eleven of them met their targeted savings and were eligible to receive their share from Medicare. However, they did improve in twenty-eight of the thirty-three quality measures, resulting in fewer falls, less tobacco usage, and better control of high blood pressure.

Shared Savings Program: The 220 ACOs in the Shared Savings Program also had trouble meeting their targets. The good news is that $300 million in savings was generated. The bad news is that only fifty-three providers beat their targets by enough to share in the savings. Another fifty-two reduced costs but didn't hit their targets. One overspent its target by $10 million.[19]

However, many providers reported that they are moving to ACOs with commercial insurers or Medicare Advantage programs, because their requirements are less complex. Although this is a disappointment for the government program, it does boost the ACO concept. The pilot also gave the providers more experience in running ACOs.[20]

Five Other Integrated Care Models

The Accountable Care Organization is the most popular integrated care model being tested. The ACA also directed the CMS Innovation Center to develop and test other models. You may hear about one of these at your next doctor or hospital visit. Here are five other innovative integrated care models that are being tested.

Bundled Payments: Medicare pays providers a targeted amount for an entire episode of care, such as a heart attack, hip replacement, or stroke. Payment of a targeted amount takes the place of the traditional fee-for-service model where Medicare pays for each test, procedure, or surgery involved. It should also not be confused with the population-based model, mentioned earlier in the chapter, which pays a set amount for each patient in the ACO.

Bundled payments would standardize payments for each procedure. According to a recent study, Medicare payments for common surgeries varied as much as 40 percent among hospitals, even those in similar areas and that provide the same level of care. Hospitals also vary greatly in the care they provide after discharge. If this were standardized, it would provide better care for the patient and lower costs for Medicare. That's important because half of all Medicare's non-drug spending went toward care that occurred during hospital stays or within ninety days of discharge.

Bundled payments encourage the hospital to coordinate care, reduce duplication, and to lower actual costs so that they come in below the bundled payment cost. The following four pilot programs began on January 31, 2013, and run until 2016.

1. **Hospital stay only.** Medicare pays a discounted fee for hospital services during a stay. If the hospital can provide the same level of care for a lower cost, it keeps the difference.

2. **Hospital stay plus aftercare.** Medicare pays a discounted fee for the hospital stay, plus either thirty, sixty, or ninety days of aftercare.

3. **Aftercare only.** Medicare pays a discounted fee for aftercare provided by a nursing home, rehab facility, long-term care facility, or home health agency. The care must begin within thirty days of the hospital stay and can be for thirty, sixty, or ninety days.

4. **All services provided during the hospital stay.** Medicare pays a discounted fee to the hospital for its services, plus those provided by other doctors and practitioners while the patient is in the hospital. This includes extra payments to cover any readmissions. If the patient doesn't need to be readmitted, the hospital increases its profit. In other words, the hospital makes more money if it keeps the patient healthy. [21]

Overall, the bundled payments program has been well-received. There were 2,412 providers that signed up in the first year. That number tripled in 2014 when another 4,122 medical groups and hospitals got on board. By 2016, a majority of health-care providers expect to implement bundled payment contracts. [22]

Partnership for Patients: The ACA granted $1 billion to hospitals and organizations that enrolled in the Partnership for Patients. It seeks to achieve its goals over three years.

The Partnership's first goal is to reduce hospital-acquired conditions, such as bedsores, blood clots from surgery, and infections, by 40 percent. It has funded twenty-six organizations, working with 3,700 hospitals, to achieve this goal. For example, most infections can be prevented by doctors and medical professionals washing their hands in between seeing each patient. However, busy doctors and nurses often forget this important task.

Hand-washing alone would eliminate 1.8 million patient injuries and save sixty thousand lives.

The Partnership's second goal is to reduce by 20 percent the number of hospital patients who are readmitted within the first thirty days after release. If successful, it would keep 1.6 million patients from returning to the hospital due to preventable conditions. In 2015, there were seventy-two community-based organizations that helped patients safely transition from the hospital to another care facility or to their own homes.[23]

Primary Care Initiative: Medicare pays a monthly fee to selected primary care doctors' offices. In return, doctors promise to provide personalized care plans for patients with chronic diseases, provide twenty-four-hour access to care and information, deliver preventive care, coordinate care with specialists, and engage patients in their own care. Medicare works with health insurance plans to support these doctors' efforts.

In 2015, there were 2,805 providers serving 404,150 Medicare/Medicaid beneficiaries. No doubt their other 2.7 million patients benefit as well. The test runs until 2016.

Primary Care Initiatives have been successful already. For example, Community Care of North Carolina reduced hospitalizations for asthma by 40 percent and visits to the emergency room by 16 percent.[24]

Federally Qualified Health Center (FQHC) Advanced Primary Care Practice Demonstration: Although the name is long and complicated, it's really just a more rigorous version of the Primary Care Initiative. The more commonly used name is patient-centered medical home, or even just medical home. These are typically community health centers that focus on Medicaid and Medicare patients.

The 434 centers receive $6 a month for each of their 195,000 Medicare patients. They are encouraged to use the funds to expand services and hours, and to focus on helping patients self-manage chronic conditions. The goal is to get these patients to think of the community health center for most of their health needs. This cuts back on their use of the hospital emergency room as their primary care physician.[25]

Medicare-Medicaid Financial Alignment Initiative: This tests two methods of coordinating care for the more than nine million Medicare recipients who also receive

Medicaid. In the Capitated model, the state and insurance companies contract with CMS to work with their health providers to deliver care more efficiently and then share the savings. In the Managed-Fee-for-Service model, the state contracts with CMS to manage efficiently on behalf of its insurance companies and health-care providers.[26]

Electronic Health Records

Although the first email was sent in 1971 and the first website created on August 6, 1991, most doctors' offices kept their medical records on paper files and faxed them when necessary.[27]

Obamacare changes that. All your medical records are being transferred from paper files to computers. Thanks to the new regulations, 78 percent of office-based doctors used electronic health records (EHRs) in 2013. The ACA's goal is for all Medicare service providers (that's nearly all doctors) to be fully functional on electronic health records by 2015.

Actually, the shift began as a carrot in the Economic Stimulus Act in 2009. More than $16.5 billion in subsidies went to hospitals and doctors who treated Medicare patients to help them transfer to EHRs. The ACA added the stick—those that didn't switch by 2015 would be penalized with lower Medicare payments.

EHRs are the base that makes the rest of health-care reform possible, including the following changes:

1. Episode-based payment.
2. Value-based purchasing.
3. A reduction in hospital readmissions.
4. Fewer hospital-acquired conditions.
5. Financial rewards for successful ACOs.[28]

EHRs also help you use technology to make management of your health care easier. You can use your phone, iPad, or computer to more easily fill prescriptions, schedule appointments, and communicate with your doctor.[29]

Probably most importantly, EHRs lower health-care costs. Over time, this lowers the cost of health insurance, especially Medicare. For more, see chapter 5.

Five Benefits of Electronic Health Records

The EHR system connects all providers and points of care. This provides the following five benefits:

1. **Enhances the efficiency of doctor appointments.** Visits can be coordinated so patients see all the different specialists at the clinic on the same day. At the very least, assistants don't have to run around between doctors carrying paper files.

2. **Makes health care safer, since records aren't lost in transit.** Hospital administrators can analyze the data to make inpatient care safer. For example, Cleveland Clinic used data analysis to find and improve infection rates. Since then, central-line infections fell 40 percent, and urinary-tract infections were also down by 40 percent. If you've ever had either, you know what a huge difference it makes to be free of them. These reductions also save lives, especially among the elderly.

3. **Makes your medical records easier for you to access.** That allows you to be in charge of managing your own health care. People are encouraged to be more responsible for their own health, and over time, costs are reduced.

These portals are modeled after the government's Blue Button that is used by Medicare and the US Department of Veterans Affairs (VA). For example, Kaiser Permanente found that doctors who switched to digital records saved the system $158,478 per every 1,000 diabetic patients. That's because better self-care meant a 5.5 percent drop in emergency room visits and a 5.3 percent decline in hospitalizations.[30]

4. **Creates a tool physicians can use to integrate services.** Doctors can quickly coordinate care with specialists, hospitals, and even mental health counselors within their system. This means that medicines aren't overprescribed and treatments don't counteract each other.

5. **Establishes a database to guide the best treatments.** Medical professionals, instead of insurance staff, can analyze the best practices of other hospitals to create

guidelines. Doctors will be able to quickly use these guidelines to decide what works best in a certain situation and what doesn't.

For example, say you have a torn rotator cuff. Your doctor doesn't think it's too bad, but just to be on the safe side, refers you for an MRI. The radiologist consults with the doctor and suggests a less expensive ultrasound instead. She bases this recommendation on evidence that the ultrasound does a better job of diagnosing the problem and costs a whole lot less. Normally, a physician wouldn't listen to a technician. The EHR provides the technician with data that allows the doctor to feel safe knowing he's not at risk of a lawsuit by ordering this less expensive procedure.

So-called big data allows hospitals and other medical systems to analyze the overall health of their patient populations. Response time is faster in response to large public health emergencies, such as seasonal flu epidemics. All this data allows hospitals to improve responsiveness. They'll track patients through their life and then compare the individuals to the general population, according to Jan De Witte, CEO of General Electric's health-care IT division.

The Pitfalls of Electronic Health Records

The next time you visit your doctor, you may notice him typing into a laptop or iPad. He's not playing computer games; he's entering notes about your visit. Unfortunately, this is making most doctors miserable. Why? They are forced to choose among 140,000 different codes to enter your diagnosis.

The administrators at the federal agencies that developed the system are excited about how they'll be able to use the data to improve diagnoses (more about that later in the chapter). But they probably didn't think enough about how it affects doctors. Nevertheless, the project rolled out on October 1, 2013.[31]

A 2014 AMA survey uncovered eight areas where doctors were demoralized by EHRs. Although the system was better than paper records, it was not user-friendly.

For example, doctors would fill out multiple boxes on forms, often entering the same information over and over again. Others found that a new patient had twenty-five different boxes checked on her record. The doctor had to talk with her, anyway, and discovered she really only had six underlying problems. He then had to enter all *that* information into new little boxes.

Doctors were the only ones who could correctly enter the data about each patient they saw. They often took paper notes during the visit, and then typed them into a system that was unwieldy and inefficient. This added to their administrative duties, taking time away from patient care.

Retrieving the records wasn't easy, either, since each network had its own system. The software was often incompatible. As a result, doctors could only retrieve records from providers in the same health-care network.[32]

Why was the system so bad? It was designed to be used for a variety of health-related users, including regulators, health insurance companies, auditors, and lawyers. As a result, it tried to be all things to all people, instead of being designed with maximizing the doctor-patient relationship.

Why can't an assistant or transcriptionist enter the records? If the information entered is incorrect, doctors may be penalized by Medicare. The value-based payment model uses this system to see if hospitals and doctors are adhering to its standards of care. Doctors can't afford to have the data be inaccurate, so they feel they must do it themselves.

Doctors must also use only certified technology. Unfortunately, the software prioritizes ease-of-use in reading the reports, not the data-entry interface. The AMA recommends that the federal certification criteria allow the EHR vendors to focus on the doctors' needs as well as those of the government.

In addition, doctors are hampered by their own corporate policies, various regulations, and even their training. The AMA plans to work with physicians, vendors, federal and state policymakers, institutions and health-care systems, and researchers to adopt its recommendations.[33]

One of the unfortunate side effects of EHR mandates is that they are driving doctors out of private practices. In 2013, only 36 percent of doctors were in private practices, down substantially from 57 percent in 2000, according to the 2012 Accenture Physicians Alignment Survey. More than half (53 percent) said the cost of electronic medical records was one reason. Nearly all (87 percent) cited overall business expenses, while 39 percent said too many patients were required in order to break even.

The cost, in both dollars and time, to install a system is frightening for small practices. In 2011, the Agency for Healthcare Research and Quality (AHRQ) found that the average initial cost is $162,000 for a five-person practice. Such a practice can expect another $85,500 for first-year maintenance costs, and 134 hours per doctor in training.

However, EHRs did improve efficiency and profits for these practices once they got past the learning curve. The Medical Group Management Association reported that the average revenue increased by nearly $50,000 per doctor, and that profits rose at least 10 percent after five years. The EHRs helped increase day-to-day efficiency, lowered transcription costs, and reduced billing errors.[34]

Big Data Analysis Comes to Health Care

Imagine walking into a hospital room in the not-too-distant future. The patient is attached to the normal tubes and wires to measure heart rate, temperature, and blood pressure. The difference is that all this data goes to an HBox that's connected to a computer network. The innovative device transfers the raw data to the hospital's EHR.

In a darkened room full of computer screens at the hub of the hospital, a handful of doctors monitor this patient and others in the hospital. The HBox allows them to monitor patients resting at home, using data transmitted from their smartphone, Fitbit, or other wearable device. The physicians compare their patients' data and conditions with similar diseases and recommend treatment plans that are stored in the hospital's computer.

This room exists, although only in prototype, at Los Angeles-based NantHealth. Its creator is Patrick Soon-Shiong, the richest doctor in the history of the world. That's because he invented Abraxane, which increased cancer survival rates by 80 percent.

The HBox can also act like the tricorder used by the fictional Dr. McCoy in *Star Trek*. It quickly takes the patient's vitals and blood tests, sending the results to computers that analyze the results, make suggested diagnoses, and recommend treatments to the doctor in real time. The patient activates apps on her cell phone to monitor her recovery, sending the data back to the doctor's computer.[35]

If this sounds too futuristic, it is—for now. But whether Dr. Soon-Shiong is successful or not, companies are headed in this direction. And it's all made possible by electronic medical records mandated by the Affordable Care Act.

According to the *MIT Technology Review*, EHRs mean that "analytic algorithms and predictive modeling mine the layers of data for patterns and insight." What does that mean for you?

You'll receive more precise and personalized diagnoses. When your health scan is combined with genomics data, for example, it allows your doctor to prescribe medication that's most effective for that gene defect.

Your doctor will use decision-support tools to recommend diagnoses and the best treatments. These tools sort through relevant research to find cases similar to yours. Your doctor still uses her own knowledge and experience, but now has access to the wisdom of her peers throughout the country.

The tools are based on sophisticated computer models that are able to analyze massive amounts of data to uncover patterns and trends. This knowledge is passed back to your doctor. It's especially helpful in diagnosing complicated cases, in avoiding risky and expensive surgeries, and in identifying new diseases.

Researchers can analyze enough data to allow new insights into disease and treatment. Genomics data allowed the Ebola virus to be tracked as it evolved throughout Africa. Analysts determined that its mutations permitted the virus to become airborne through sneezing, but not through dry dust particles.[36]

The same type of data analysis is already available to advertisers, retailers like Amazon, and online interfaces like Google, Facebook, and Pinterest. They use all kinds of intimate data to determine what you will buy, and provide more ad choices to you. Now that same kind of technology is becoming available to doctors to do something important—save lives.

What makes this possible? All types of public health information combined into one database and made accessible to those who need it most.

Right now, health-related data is spread out among the seven following sources:

1. **Insurance claims.** Maintains information about trends in disease diagnoses, prescription drug use, and success of operations for a large percentage of the population.
2. **Public health records.** Provides insights into health trends across communities from federal and state records, including Medicare, Medicaid, and the Centers for Disease Control and Preventions (CDC).
3. **Environmental.** Mapping, location, and weather data add insight into what may be affecting health in communities from geographic or weather causes.
4. **Genomic and biotech.** Genome sequencing offers detailed information on how diseases evolve and what role genetics play in diseases. For example, scientists found more than 100 genes underlying schizophrenia. With this knowledge, drug companies began researching specific medicines to target these genes.[37]
5. **Mobile health apps.** There are already 100,000 mobile health apps that measure exercise, heart rates, and diet. This includes wearable devices such as Fitbit.
6. **Family health history.** These records combine with genomic data to understand how lifestyle choices can overcome genetic predispositions.
7. **Electronic medical records.** Once computerized, the data allows analysis of lab results, prescriptions, detailed notes about appearance and behavior, and success of different treatments.

For example, IBM uses its Watson artificial intelligence computer system to help oncologists. It's part of a $1 billion effort to apply the technology that won *Jeopardy* to win the battle against cancer.

The artificial intelligence program analyzes a patient's medical records along with the latest knowledge in medical journals, textbooks, and treatment guidelines. Oncology centers use Watson to diagnose and treat lung, colorectal, and breast cancer in New York and leukemia in Texas.

Watson improves these doctors' bottom line because they don't have to refer their patients out to specialists. It may also help avoid the looming crisis in cancer care by making each doctor more effective and able to treat more patients. The American Society of Clinical Oncology reports that cancer cases will increase by 42 percent by 2025, but the number of oncologists will lag behind, rising only 28 percent.[38]

That future is why the tech experts at CMS created 140,000 different codes (actually, they only created 122,000; there were already 18,000 in use before). According to Pat Brooks, senior technical adviser at the Center, good data analysis requires this level of detail. In the long run, it improves both the accuracy of the data and the quality of care.

The Blue Button Connector

In 2014, HealthIT.gov launched the Blue Button Connector. You can use this site right now to find out which of your medical records are online. Most major health insurance companies, pharmacies, and hospitals are participants. That means most will probably use the Blue Button to connect to the data analysis systems mentioned in the previous sections. Larger companies might decide to create their own proprietary access portal.

Go to the Blue Button Connector to find out if your providers have joined yet. There are also thirty apps listed to help you manage your health-care information online. The link is bluebuttonconnector.healthit.gov/.

You can go online to make appointments, fill prescriptions, and review hospital discharge notes. Use it to update your health history online so you won't have to show up fifteen minutes early at your next appointment to fill out the same paperwork you did last year.

In the next few years, you'll be able to go online to review test results, manage and fill in daily records for diabetes and other chronic conditions, and even download your fitness results from the gym's treadmill to your doctor's office.

These online health records will be especially helpful, for example, if your child has an accident while away from home and has to go to the emergency room. You'll be able to review your own health-care history from the hospital where you were born, to your pediatrician, and on up to your current doctor.

Value-Based Health Care: What Is It?

Christine Dayton was diagnosed with Stage 3 ovarian cancer, where the statistics are "very scary," she said. Fortunately, she was successful in fighting the cancer. However, the grueling chemotherapy, surgery, and radiation treatment left her with neuropathy. She lost feeling in her hands and wondered what to do next.

That's where the Palliative Care Program stepped in. Palliative comes from the Latin word meaning "to cloak," and its goal is to wrap the patient in a cloak of relief from the symptoms, pain, and stress of serious illnesses like cancer. This program coordinated all the care for Christine, and the cancer went into remission. However, the program didn't stop there. It coordinated follow-up care for her neuropathy. It found counseling to help Christine with the emotional impact the cancer had on her and her four boys. The doctor also advised her on the wisdom of having a double mastectomy, since ovarian cancer is highly likely to spread. [39]

As mentioned in the section on ACOs, one of the key cornerstones of health-care reform is switching from fee-for-service to bundled payments. Why is the payment system so important?

Nearly 80 percent of Medicare and two-thirds of Medicaid payments followed the fee-for-service model. It seems pretty straightforward since this is how you pay for everything from gasoline to glasses to groceries. You pay for what you get. However, the grocery clerk or the gas station attendant doesn't tell you how much you need to buy. Doctors do. We rely on their expertise to decide whether we need a colonoscopy, back surgery, or MRI.

That system isn't a problem when it's obvious, such as setting a broken bone or receiving antibiotics for pneumonia. However, it can get a little dicey when the diagnosis and remedy are not as clear. If you have back pain, do you need physical therapy, painkillers, or surgery? Should a baby be delivered naturally or by cesarean section? Do you really need that hip replacement now?

If you think your doctor is 100 percent right on every decision, think again. When forty cardiologists were surveyed about whether a patient with a certain set of symptoms should have surgery, 50 percent said yes and 50 percent said no. Two years later, they repeated the survey, and this time 40 percent of the cardiologists had changed their minds.[40]

Fee-for-service created a fragmented system where each service, test, or procedure was billed separately to Medicare, Medicaid, and health insurance companies. This inadvertently rewarded volume over value and is one of the contributing factors in higher health-care costs.

Most of the past remedies focused on across-the-board pay cuts. Capitation meant the doctor would receive a set fee per month per patient, regardless of services provided. Managed care organizations used capitation to cut costs, and reviewed the doctors' care to make sure shortcuts weren't taken. The doctor took all the risk, and so naturally capitation wasn't very popular.[41]

Instead, the ACA requires Medicare switch to value-based payments. Doctors who provide higher value care will receive higher payments than those who provide lower quality care. HHS announced in January 2015 that Medicare will switch half of all non-managed care to value-based payments by 2018.

They also have to meet performance measurements or they will be docked pay. That means doctors will have financial incentives to work toward better patient outcomes. These outcomes will be actually measured, so they'll get paid more for quicker recoveries, fewer readmissions, lower infection rates, and fewer medical errors. That's the value in value-based payments.

The top health-care providers already proved this works. For example, the Cleveland Clinic recognized a long time ago that coordinated care led to better results with lower costs. As a result, it put doctors on staff and paid them with one-year contracts that held them accountable for outcomes, as well as performing research. The other advantage was that by having all the doctors on the same team, it was much easier to coordinate care—especially if all doctors were paid by the same method.

The Clinic uses bundled payments within its own system. Bundled payments reimburse hospitals, doctors, and providers a flat rate for each episode of care, regardless of how many tests or procedures are ordered. For example, the cost of a hip replacement is known up front, even if complications arise. Studies in hospitals show this is more efficient and eliminates duplicate or unnecessary tests, but does not cut back on care. The savings are shared between providers and the Medicare program.

The Cleveland Clinic also created care centers that each focus on one specialty. These "institutes" combine medical and surgical departments that specialize in treating one disease or part of the body. The center receives one payment for, say, a hip replacement. If it can reduce the costs through coordinating care, it shares the savings with the Clinic.

The Clinic lowered costs more than $150 million by cutting its supply expenses. It uses data analysis of electronic health records to get the best price, negotiate better contracts, and replace supplies with competitive parts of equal value.

HMOs, like those run by Kaiser Permanente and Humana, also use bundled payments. They already treat 30 percent of the fifty-four million Medicare beneficiaries.[42]

The ACA requires Medicare to pay hospitals based on how well they perform in quality of care. Hospitals will set up systems to comply. Over time, that means doctors, and ultimately insurance companies, will follow. In other words, doctors must prove that treatment resulted in better care and fewer return visits. This will result in better follow-up care from hospitals and help them shift to helping people take better care of themselves.[43]

Value-Based Payments Is Based on Quantifiable Metrics

CMS pays based on how well a hospital follows certain metrics that measure high quality and higher value.

The Hospital Readmissions Reduction Program began on October 1, 2012. It attempts to prevent the problems that cause patients to have to return to the hospital within thirty days after they are discharged. Hospital readmissions cause unnecessary suffering to patients and their families, and significantly increase health-care spending.[44]

The program focuses on three conditions that either frequently cause readmissions or have a significant cost when they occur. These are heart attacks, heart failure, and pneumonia. If a hospital has above-average readmissions, its Medicare payments are lowered.

Sometimes the readmission is something the hospital couldn't have done anything about. Patients might have complications from the procedure like infections or drug interactions. Or the disease might suddenly take a turn for the worse.

Other times, the hospital should have done more. For example, patients might not have received good treatment while at the hospital. Or their aftercare was inadequate: They didn't receive thorough follow-up care instructions, didn't take their medications correctly, and then got dizzy and fell.

It looks like the program is working already. In 2013, CMS reported that hospital readmission rates dropped by 130,000 between January 2012 and August 2013.[45]

The Hospital Value-Based Purchasing (VBP) Program, which began in Fiscal Year 2013, is basically pay-for-performance for inpatient stays. It measures levels of care using hospital statistics and patient surveys. In 2015, 3,500 hospitals agreed to participate.

The hospitals were ranked on how well they followed the basics of care for the riskiest patients. This accounted for nearly half (45 percent) of the total score. It measured things like whether heart attack patients were given discharge instructions, whether heart surgery patients had their urinary catheters removed within two days after surgery, and how often patients with pneumonia had their blood culture analyzed so they could be given the right antibiotic.

These seem pretty straightforward, and you'd hope they were always done. It's easy to see how, if they weren't, it would cause pretty severe complications.

Hospital pay was also partially determined by whether patients felt cared for. A survey was given to a sample of patients between forty-eight hours and six weeks after discharge that was worth 30 percent of the total score. Patients were asked if they felt their nurses and doctors always communicated well. They were also asked whether the nurses explained things clearly, listened carefully, and treated them with courtesy and respect.

Patients were also asked whether they felt the hospital staff was always responsive to their needs. For example, did they respond quickly when patients used the call button?

Other questions asked whether pain was always controlled, was the hospital always clean and quiet at night, and if staff always explained the medicines that were administered. If you've ever stayed at a hospital, you know how important all these issues are in making sure you get well quickly. Find more detail on the actual survey at www.medicare.gov/hospitalcompare/Data/Overview.html.

The final area of measurement is whether the most vulnerable patients—those who had heart attacks, heart failure, or pneumonia—die within the thirty days after being admitted to the hospital. This measurement is worth 25 percent of the total score.

After these percentages are totaled, the hospital is given four scores. The achievement score is based on how well the hospital followed the specific procedures, while the improvement score measures how much the hospital has improved. The third score compares the hospital to others in its class. The fourth score is weighted to boost the achievement or improvement score, whichever is higher.

Best of all, these scores are available to the public at Medicare's Hospital Compare Site, at www.medicare.gov/hospitalcompare/search.html. You can use this information when shopping for health insurance plans or when comparing hospitals for an elective procedure.

The ACA Pays Doctors to Coordinate Care of the Chronically Ill

In 2014, the ACA added another component. It began paying doctors to coordinate care for Medicare patients with chronic conditions. These seniors often received disjointed and fragmented care that was difficult for them to manage themselves. For example, sometimes they'd show up for an appointment, but the tests hadn't been delivered yet, and no one really knew why they were there.

Doctors draft and execute a comprehensive plan for patients with two or more chronic conditions. These typically include heart disease, diabetes, and depression. While two-thirds of Medicare beneficiaries fall into this category, they create 93 percent of Medicare costs.

Signing up for this care gives patients twenty-four-hour access to health providers to advise them on urgent conditions. This helps keep them out of the hospital emergency room.

As part of the coordinated care, doctors agree to look at not just the patients' medical needs, but their psychological and social needs as well. Doctors check to make sure these patients are taking all of their medicine correctly and even monitor the care provided by other doctors. Most importantly, they assume responsibility for making sure patients receive follow-up care once they leave the hospital. In return, Medicare pays the doctors $42 a month for each patient, who provide a 20 percent co-pay for the service.

The Blueprint for Insurance Companies Is Value-Based Payments

Health insurance companies are also being affected by the value-based payment model. For example, the ACA's requirement that companies pay 100 percent for all preventive care is actually a form of value-based payment. That's because preventive care has been shown to lower health-care costs and increase patient wellness across the board.

The ACA encourages the HHS and the Department of Labor to begin a conversation with insurance companies, business groups, and medical associations on the best way to encourage value-based payments in more insurance plans.

As a result, many employers have begun switching to value-based payments. For example, the insurance for the public employees in the state of Oregon pays more for preventive care, medications for chronic disease, and true emergencies. It pays less for procedures where a cheaper, yet successful, option is available. For example, a doctor gets reimbursed less for a back surgery if physical therapy hasn't been tried. Patients who smoke pay $25 more in premiums a month, while patients who go to Weight Watchers can bring their spouses for free.[46]

Is It Working?

Hospital executives have renewed their focus on excellence in the areas that Medicare measures. For example, some hospitals have reduced nighttime noise—one of the questions patients are asked about—by replacing squeaky wheels on food carts and discouraging hospital staff from chatting on cell phones outside of patients' rooms.

Others redouble their efforts to ensure heart attack patients always get an angioplasty within ninety minutes of arrival, another area that is scored. Some private insurers have adopted similar incentives.[47]

Some doctors decided that the money isn't worth it. Dr. Mathew Press reported in the *New England Journal of Medicine* what it took to coordinate the care of a seventy-year old man with bile duct liver cancer. Over the course of nearly three months, Dr. Press coordinated eleven office visits and five procedures with ten doctors. He talked to these doctors forty times and the patient or his wife twelve times.[48]

Dr. Mark Sklar, with the George Washington University Medical Center, must reduce the number of written prescriptions handed to patients by contacting the pharmacy directly. If he doesn't reach the goal mandated by the ACA regulations, his Medicare reimbursements can be cut as much as 5 percent.

However, Medicare patients aren't comfortable with the digital age. They're used to paper prescriptions and resist the doctor's attempts to comply with Medicare. Who does Dr. Sklar serve—the US government or his patients?

Similarly, the Physician Quality Reporting System requires Dr. Sklar to enter data complying with nine codes for every visit. These include quality of care measurements such as blood pressure and blood sugar levels. Although this benefits the patient, it also means the doctor must spend more time in front of the computer, entering codes. To comply, the doctor must cut back on his personal weekend time.[49]

How You Benefit

Customer service and how you're treated are things you take for granted when using most services. You wouldn't return to a grocery store that wasn't clean or where the staff was too busy to help you. Yet with hospitals, you often don't have a choice. Sometimes it's the only one in the area. Other times, you're in an emergency situation. Often, it's the most highly rated hospital for your particular procedure. More likely than not, it's the only one your insurance plan covers.

That's what's so different about health care. You often don't get a chance to shop, price compare, and do the research you'd do when buying a car. You generally don't even know what the price is—since the insurance company pays for it. Or, if you don't have insurance, you can't afford it, no matter who offers the best price.

That's why it's good when the federal government steps in to protect you. With the Value-Based Payment Program, the hospitals know they get docked in pay if they don't treat you well. Most people have no idea that Obamacare is doing this for them.

In addition to the Hospital Compare website mentioned previously, Medicare offers the Guide to Choosing a Hospital. You can download it at www.medicare.gov/Pubs/pdf/10181 .pdf.

Even if you never go to the hospital, the Value-Based Purchasing Program helps you by lowering overall health-care costs. A reduction in hospital-acquired diseases could save $4 billion annually, while fewer hospital readmissions could save as much as $26 billion each year. In total, Value-Based Purchasing is expected to reduce Medicare spending by $214 billion over the next ten years. That translates to lower premiums, not to mention a safer hospital stay, for you and your family.[50]

Three Ways Obamacare Is Already Successful

The ACA is already having a powerful impact on the cost of health care by slowing its rate of growth. The ACA has also had a similar impact on the rate of increases in health insurance and Medicare costs. On top of that, the ACA lowers payments to medical providers and Medicare Advantage insurance companies directly. This further slows the growth rate of Medicare costs. Last but not least, the costs of implementing the ACA itself are less than was originally projected.

The Cost of Health Care Is Rising, But at a Slower Rate

Between 1990 and 2008, health-care costs rose 7.2 percent each year, twice the pace of economic growth.

From 2009 to 2012 they rose 4.2 percent a year, thanks to the financial crisis and recession. However, even though the recession is over, the cost of health care is still rising at a slower rate than before. CMS projected it would rise 5.76 percent a year from 2013 through 2023.[51]

That's why President Obama said, "Health-care spending has risen more slowly than at any time in the last forty years."[52]

In January 2015, UnitedHealth Group, the largest health insurer in the nation, reported better-than-expected earnings, thanks to lower medical costs. It pointed to the success of the ACA's Value-Based Payment Program. Thanks to this success, it expanded its offerings on the exchanges from four to twenty-four. As a result, it serviced 88.5 million people at the end of 2014, compared to 88.2 million the year before.[53]

Medicare Cost Increases Are Moderating

The growth of Medicare spending is also slowing. In 2012, it grew 4.0 percent, followed by 3.4 percent growth in 2013, thanks to the ACA and sequestration. CMS projected 4.2 percent growth in 2014, slowing to 2.7 percent growth in 2015, thanks to lower payments to Medicare Advantage. From 2016 through 2023, CMS forecasts 7.3 percent annual growth, thanks to the compounded effects of an aging population of Baby Boomers.

This coincides with estimates by the CBO. In 2010, it projected that Medicare spending would rise to $12,376 per beneficiary by 2014, and $14,913 by 2019. Instead, spending fell by $1,209 a person, to $11,167 by 2014. The CBO also forecast costs to rise to just $12,478 per beneficiary by 2019.[54]

That means the Medicare Hospital Insurance Trust Fund won't run out of money until 2023. That's four years later than projected last year, and thirteen years later than projected in 2009, the year before the ACA passed. As a result, Medicare Part B premiums will stay at $104.90 a month—the same as the past three years.

What happened? The Kaiser Family Foundation gave five reasons:

1. The ACA reduced payments to providers and to Medicare Advantage plans. That's because costs for administering Parts A and B were rising 9.2 percent, much faster than the government's own costs. Many experts felt these companies were simply overcharging the government. Insurance companies were OK with the reduced payments because the mandate would send them more customers. For more on the mandate, see chapter 8.

2. Medicare began rolling out accountable care organizations, bundled payments, and value-based payments. As a result, spending on hospital care hasn't risen since 2011. For example, hospital readmissions dropped by 150,000 in 2012 and then again in 2013.

3. In 2013, high-income earners paid more in Medicare payroll taxes, as well as Medicare Part B and D premiums.

4. That same year, Congress imposed spending cuts known as sequestration. This lowered Medicare payments to providers and plans by 2 percent.

5. Drug costs have dropped because several expensive, brand-name drugs have gone off patent. At the same time, insurance companies are switching to generics in their formularies wherever possible.[55]

Obamacare Costs Are Lower Than Expected

Surprise! Premiums on the health-care exchanges are actually *lower* than the CBO originally projected. That's because the CBO expected that people would choose plans that were just as comprehensive as those offered by employers. Instead, people are choosing plans that have smaller networks, offer fewer health-care services, and pay less to doctors and hospitals. The premiums are lower than expected because people are buying plans that are more cost-efficient. Now that they have a chance to shop, they want the plan with the lowest price tag. The powerful competitive force of the free market will continue driving down insurance and health-care costs.

As a result, the average 2014 premium for the benchmark Silver plan was $317 a month, increasing to $325 a month in 2015. By 2016, the premium will be 15 percent lower than originally anticipated. Lower premiums means lower subsidies, since they are based on the average cost of the Silver plan. That means Obamacare will cost taxpayers $61 billion less over the next ten years.[56]

In the near term, however, insurance companies in some states (including New Mexico, Tennessee, and Maryland) sought 25 percent to 50 percent rate increases in 2015. They claimed the ACA increased their health-care costs as new enrollees received treatment for heretofore undiagnosed illnesses. Although that might be true in some specific areas, costs across the board haven't risen as much.[57]

The Real Reason Your Health-Care Costs Are Higher

In a 2014 Kaiser poll, 60 percent of Americans said that health-care costs are going up faster than usual in recent years. Most of them blame Obamacare. However, as we just saw, the ACA is lowering the cost of health care. Why do people think costs are rising, then?

Nearly 150 million people get their insurance through their employers, who are pushing a greater *share* of costs onto them. Unknown to most workers, businesses have been shifting the rising cost of group plans onto their employees for years.

One way is by raising deductibles. In 2006, 45 percent of workers had a plan with no deductible. By 2014, that number had fallen to 20 percent. The average deductible more than doubled during that time period, from $584 per person to $1,217 for a single coverage plan.[58]

Why? It was coupled with the growth of Health Savings Accounts (HSA), which allowed beneficiaries to save pretax dollars to use later for medical expenses. The gains on the money invested are tax-exempt, as are the withdrawals—as long as they are used for health-care costs.

In 1996, Congress approved the tax status of these plans. In 2003, it raised the amount you could save, but only if it was tied to a high-deductible plan. The idea was to encourage people to pay for more of their own health care, so they would have more of an incentive to stay healthy.

However, that's not exactly what happened. The Government Accountability Office found that the average taxable income for HSA account holders was $139,000—more than double the average income for all taxpayers. They were using these accounts as tax-advantaged savings accounts.

Insurers used the congressional approval of high-deductible plans to push them onto businesses as a way to save money. By 2007, 6.1 million Americans had high-deductible plans, but only a small percentage also took advantage of the HSAs. That's simply because they couldn't afford them. Studies revealed that most people took the high-deductible plans, not to take advantage of the HSAs, but in order to get any coverage at all. Many of those people had preexisting conditions that regular insurance providers wouldn't cover. Others simply couldn't afford a low-deductible plan.[59]

Companies also shifted the cost of premiums onto workers. Employee share of premium cost rose from 26.7 percent in 2004 to 28.7 percent in 2014. At the same time, the total costs of premiums nearly doubled (from $9,950 in 2004 to $16,834 in 2014). As a result, the average cost of a family plan rose from $2,661 to $4,823 during that same time period.[60]

Therefore, even though Obamacare is successful in lowering health-care and health insurance costs overall, you might not feel it because companies are shifting a greater percentage of the cost onto you.

In addition, wages haven't risen at the same rate as premiums. As a result, workers see a greater chunk of their paycheck being eaten up by health insurance premiums. Premiums in 2013 rose 5 percent for singles, and 4 percent for family coverage. At the same time, average incomes only rose 1.8 percent and inflation was nearly flat, rising just 1.1 percent.

To be more than fair, companies are taking steps to lower health and insurance costs by keeping their employees healthier. For example, 74 percent of companies that provide health insurance offer at least one wellness program. One-third of the companies offer health risk assessments, with many of them offering a $500 bonus to complete the assessment.[61]

Chapter 3: References

1. Tom Tzostak, Healthcare Economics Manager, "The ABCs of ACOs," Toshiba Medical. https://www.youtube.com/watch?v=zQIf2ggEp6s, accessed August 28, 2014.

2. Elizabeth Miller Coyne, "The Disney Take on Big Data's Value," The New IP, January 13, 2015. http://www.thenewip.net/document.asp?doc_id=713004&site=thenewip, accessed May 24, 2015.

3. Toby Cosgrove, "Value-Based Healthcare Is Inevitable and That's Good," *Harvard Business Review,* September 24, 2013. http://blogs.hbr.org/2013/09/value-based-health-care-is-inevitable-and-thats-good/, accessed November 12, 2014.

4. "ACOs: Coordinated Care," Centers for Medicare and Medicaid Services, June 24, 2014. https://www.youtube.com/watch?v=9t5SDPfu5Kk&feature

5. Kim Parker and Eileen Patten, "The Sandwich Generation," Pew Research, January 30, 2013. http://www.pewsocialtrends.org/2013/01/30/the-sandwich-generation/, accessed November 10, 2014. Lynn Feinberg, Susan C. Reinhard, Ari Houser, and Rita Choula, "Valuing the Invaluable: 2011 Update," AARP Public Policy Institute, July 2011. http://assets.aarp.org/rgcenter/ppi/ltc/i51-caregiving.pdf, accessed November 10, 2014. "Family Caregivers--What They Spend, What They Sacrifice," Evercare, November 2007. http://www.caregiving.org/data/Evercare_NAC_CaregiverCost StudyFINAL20111907.pdf, accessed November 10, 2014.

6. Marilyn Werber Serafini, "The Parent Trap: Adult Children Care for Elderly Parents," Kaiser Health News, March 1, 2012. http://kaiserhealthnews.org/news/parent-trap/, accessed November 10, 2014. "Medicaid's Assisted Living Benefits: Availability and Eligability," Paying for Senior Care, April 2015. http://www.payingfor seniorcare.com/medicaid-waivers/assisted-living.html, accessed May 23, 2015.

7. "Medicaid's Assisted Living Benefits: Availability and Eligibility," Paying for Senior Care, April 2015. http://www.payingforseniorcare.com/medicaid-waivers/assisted-living.html#title2, accessed May 24, 2015.

8. "Collaboration Is the Secret Ingredient for a Solid Partnership," Anthem Press Release, July 10, 2014. http://bcbs.com/healthcare-news/plans/collaboration-is-the-secret-ingredient-for-a-solid-partnership.html, accessed November 12, 2014.

9. "Accountable Care Organizations," Medicare.gov. http://www.medicare.gov/manage-your-health/coordinating-your-care/accountable-care-organizations.html, accessed May 24, 2015.

10. "Methodology for Determining Shared Savings and Losses under the Medicare Shared Savings Program,"Medicare Learning Network,April 2014. http://www.cms.gov/Medicare/Medicare-Fee-for-Service-Payment/sharedsavingsprogram/Downloads/ACO_Methodology_Factsheet_ICN907405.pdf, accessed May 25, 2015.

11. "Fast Facts," Medicare.gov, April 2015. http://www.cms.gov/Medicare/Medicare-Fee-for-Service-Payment/sharedsavingsprogram/Downloads/All-Starts-MSSP-ACO.pdf, accessed May 25, 2015.

12. "Advance Payment ACO Model," CMS.gov. http://innovation.cms.gov/initiatives/Advance-Payment-ACO-Model/, accessed May 25, 2015.

13. "Pioneer ACO Program Frequently Asked Questions," Partners Healthcare, November 2014.

14. "Pioneer ACO Model, CMS.gov. http://innovation.cms.gov/initiatives/Pioneer-ACO-Model/, accessed May 25, 2015.

15. Jacqueline DiChiara, "Pioneer ACO Model: The Embrace of Population-Based Payments," RevCycle Intelligence, May 5, 2015. http://revcycleintelligence.com/news/pioneer-aco-model-the-embrace-of-population-based-payments, accessed May 25, 2015.

16. "Accountable Care Organizations," Health Affairs, August 13, 2010. http://www.healthaffairs.org/healthpolicybriefs/brief.php?brief_id=23, accessed May 25, 2015.

17. "The ABCs of ACOs," Toshiba Medical. http://www.youtube.com/watch?v=zQIf2ggEp6s.

18. Jordan Rau, "Nearly 1,500 Hospitals Penalized Under Medicare Program Rating Quality," Kaiser Health News, November 14, 2013. http://www.kaiserhealthnews.org/Stories/2013/November/14/value-based-purchasing-medicare.aspx, accessed November 12, 2014.

19. Melinda Beck, "A Medicare Program Loses More Healthcare Providers," *Wall Street Journal*, September 25, 2014. http://online.wsj.com/articles/a-medicare-program-loses-more-health-care-providers-1411685388, accessed November 12, 2014.

20. Mark Sklar, MD, "Doctoring in the Age of Obamacare," *Wall Street Journal*, September 12, 2014.

21. "Bundled Payments for Care Improvement (BPCI) Initiative," CMS.gov. http://innovation.cms.gov/initiatives/bundled-payments/, accessed May 25, 2015.

22. "Thousands of Providers Join Medicare's Bundled Pay Program," The Advisory Board Company, August 1, 2014. http://www.advisory.com/daily-briefing/2014/08/01/providers-join-medicare-bundled-pay-program-what-it-means/, accessed May 25, 2015.

23. "About the Partnership for Patients," CMS.gov. http://partnershipforpatients.cms.gov/about-the-partnership/aboutthepartnershipforpatients.html, accessed May 25, 2015. "Community-based Care Transitions Program," CMS.gov. http://innovation.cms.gov/initiatives/CCTP/index.html, accesssed June 17, 2015.

24. "Comprehensive Primary Care Initiative Fact Sheet," Centers for Medicare and Medicaid Innovation. http://innovation.cms.gov/initiatives/comprehensive-primary-care-initiative/ and http://www.medicare.gov/forms-help-and-resources/mail-about-medicare/comprehensive-primary-care-initiative-notice.html, accessed June 17, 2015.

25. "FQHC Advanced Primary Care Practice Demonstration," CMS.gov. http://innovation.cms.gov/initiatives/fqhcs/, accessed November 12, 2014.

26. "The Affordable Care Act: Helping Providers Help Patients," Centers for Medicare and Medicaid Services. http://www.cms.gov/Medicare/Medicare-Fee-for-Service-Payment/ACO/Downloads/ACO-Menu-Of-Options.pdf, accessed November 12, 2014.

27. Alyson Shontell, "The First Ever Email, the First Tweet, and Ten Other Famous Internet Firsts," *Business Insider*, April 23, 2013. http://finance.yahoo.com/news/the-first-ever-email—the-first-tweet—and-12-other-famous-internet-firsts-181209886.html, accessed October 9, 2014.

28. "The ABCs of ACOs," Toshiba Medical.

29. "NCHS Data: Answering the Nation's Health Questions," Centers for Disease Control and Prevention, February 2014. http://www.cdc.gov/nchs/data/factsheets/factsheet_nchs_data.htm, accessed October 9, 2014.

30. Suzanne Allard Levingston, "Electronic Health Records 'Make or Break Year'," *Bloomberg Businessweek*, November 14, 2013. http://www.businessweek.com/articles/2013-11-14/2014-outlook-electronic-health-records-make-or-break-year, accessed October 9, 2014.

31. Anna Wilde Mathews, "Walked Into a Lamppost? Help Is On the Way," *Wall Street Journal*, September 13, 2011.

32. Steve Denning, "Why Is Your Doctor Typing? Electronic Medical Records Run Amok," *Forbes*, April 25, 2013. http://www.forbes.com/sites/stevedenning/2013/04/25/why-is -your-doctor-typing-hint-think-agile/, accessed October 9, 2014.

33. "AMA Calls for Design Overhaul of Electronic Health Records to Improve Usability," American Medical Association, Sept. 16, 2014. http://www.ama-assn.org/ama/pub/ news/news/2014/2014-09-16-solutions-to-ehr-systems.page, accessed October 9, 2014.

34. Lucia DiVenere, MA, "The Affordable Care Act and the Drive for Electronic Health Records: Are Small Practices Being Squeezed?" *OBG Management*, July 2013, Vol. 26 No. 7, pages 36-44. http://www.jfponline.com/fileadmin/qhi/obg/pdfs/0713 _PDFs/0713_OBG_DiVenere.pdf, accessed June 17, 2015.

35. Matthew Herper, "Medicines' Manhattan Project," *Forbes*, September 29, 2014.

36. Richard Preston, "The Ebola Wars: How Genomics Research Can Help Contain the Outbreak," *The New Yorker*, October 27, 2014.

37. Damian Paletta, "Falling Costs Boost Medicare Outlook," *Wall Street Journal,* July 29, 2014.

38. "IBM Aims to Make Medical Expertise a Commodity," *MIT Technology Review*, Volume 117, No. 5.

39. "Palliative Medicine," Care Coordination in Fort Dodge, http://www.unitypoint.org/ fortdodge/aco-patient-testimonials.aspx

40. "More Phones, Fewer Doctors," *MIT Technology Review*, Vol. 177, No. 5.

41. Patrick C. Alguire, MD, FACP, "Understanding Capitation," American College of Physicians. http://www.acponline.org/residents_fellows/career_counseling/understandcapit. htm, accessed October 25, 2014.

42. Melanie Evans and Paul Demko, "Medicare's Payment Reform Push Draws Praise and Fears," *Modern Health Care*, January 26, 2015. http://www.modernhealthcare .com/article/20150126/NEWS/301269813, accessed June 23, 2015. Robert Pear, "Medicare to Start Paying Doctors Who Coordinate Needs of Chronically Ill Patients," *New York Times*, August 16, 2014. http://www.nytimes.com/2014/08/17/us/ medicare-to-start-paying-doctors-who-coordinate-needs-of-chronically-ill-patients .html, accessed August 28, 2014.

43. Alguire, "Understanding Capitation."

44. "Hospital Readmissions Reduction Program," Medicare.gov. http://www.medicare.gov/ hospitalcompare/readmission-reduction-program.html, accessed August 28, 2014.

45. "New Data Shows Affordable Care Act Reforms Are Leading to Lower Hospital Readmission Rates for Medicare Beneficiaries," Blogs CMS, December 6, 2013. http:// blog.cms.gov/2013/12/06/new-data-shows-affordable-care-act-reforms-are-leading-to-lower-hospital-readmission-rates-for-medicare-beneficiaries/, accessed November 12, 2104.

46. "Value-Based Insurance Design," National Conference of State Legislatures, February 2014. http://www.ncsl.org/research/health/value-based-insurance-design.aspx, accessed December 8, 2014.

47. Jordan Rau, "When TLC Doesn't Satisfy Patients, Elite Hospitals May Pay a Price," Kaiser Health News, November 7, 2011. http://kaiserhealthnews.org/news/patient-ratings-hospital-medicare-reimbursements/, accessed November 12, 2014.

48. Pear, "Medicare to Start Paying Doctors."

49. Mark Sklar, MD, "Doctoring in the Age of Obamacare," *Wall Street Journal*, September 12, 2014.

50. "Healthcare Reform Navigation: Value-Based Purchasing," *Repertoire Magazine*, September 8, 2014. http://www.repertoiremag.com/healthcare-reform-navigation-value-based-purchasing.html, accessed November 13, 2014.

51. "Study Finds Recent Slowdown in Health Spending Growth Mostly Tied to the Economy," Kaiser Family Foundation, April 22, 2013. http://kff.org/health-reform/ press-release/study-finds-recent-slowdown-in-health-spending-growth-mostly-tied-to-the-economy/, accessed June 17, 2015. "National Health Expenditures Projections 2013-2023," CMS. http://www.cms.gov/Research-Statistics-Data-and-Systems/ Statistics-Trends-and-Reports/NationalHealthExpendData/Downloads/Proj2013. pdf, accessed June 17, 2015.

52. Mark Landler and Michael D. Shear, "Enrollments Exceed Obama's Target for Healthcare Act," *New York Times*, April 17, 2014. http://www.nytimes.com/2014/04/18/ us/obama-says-young-adults-push-health-care-enrollment-above-targets.html, accessed September 3, 2014.

53. Anna Wilde Mathews and Michael Calia, "UnitedHealth Benefits From Medical Cost Trends," *Wall Street Journal*, January 22, 2015.

54. "National Health Expenditures 2013 Highlights," CMS. http://www.cms.gov/Research-Statistics-Data-and-Systems/Statistics-Trends-and-Reports/National HealthExpendData/Downloads/highlights.pdf, accessed June 17, 2015. "National Health Expenditure Projections 2013-2023," CMS. http://www.cms.gov/Research-Statistics-Data-and-Systems/Statistics-Trends-and-Reports/NationalHealth ExpendData/Downloads/highlights.pdf, accessed June 17, 2015. David Lawder, "U.S. Healthcare Spending to Slow Further: Government Report," Reuters, September 3, 2014. http://www.reuters.com/article/2014/09/03/us-usa-healthcare-spending-idUS KBN0GY2I620140903, accessed September 3, 2014. Julie Rovner, "Good News for Boomers, Medicare's Hospital Trust Fund Appears Flush Until 2030," Kaiser Health News, July 28, 2014. http://kaiserhealthnews.org/news/medicare-trustees -say-fund-will-last-until-2030/, accessed September 2, 2014.

55. Trisha Neuman and Julietter Cubanski, "The Mystery of the Missing $1,200 per Person: Can Medicare's Spending Slowdown Continue?" Kaiser Family Foundation Perspectives, September 29, 2014. http://kff.org/health-costs/perspective/the-mystery -of-the-missing-1000-per-person-can-medicares-spending-slowdown-continue/, accessed June 17, 2015.

56. Jason Millman, "Lower Premiums (Yes, Really) Drive Down Obamacare's Expected Costs, CBO Says," *Washington Post*, April 14, 2014. http://www.washingtonpost.com/ blogs/wonkblog/wp/2014/04/14/lower-premiums-yes-really-drive-down-obamacares -expected-costs-cbo-says/, accessed June 17, 2015.

57. Louise Radnofsky, "Health Insurers Seek Hefty Rate Boosts," *Wall Street Journal*, May 21, 2015. http://www.wsj.com/articles/health-insurers-seek-hefty-rate-boosts -1432244042, accessed May 26, 2015.

58. "2014 Employer Health Benefits Survey," Kaiser Family Foundation, September 10, 2014. http://kff.org/report-section/ehbs-2014-summary-of-findings/, accessed June 17, 2015.

59. Michael Hiltzik, "High Deductibles and Obamacare Derangement Syndrome," *Los Angeles Times*, March 11, 2014. http://articles.latimes.com/2014/mar/11/business/ la-fi-mh-obamacare-derangement-20140311, accessed September 6, 2014. Michael Hiltzik, "Shedding Risk: Insurers See Banking Future," *Los Angeles Times*, October 22, 2008. https://s3.amazonaws.com/s3.documentcloud.org/documents/1076511/ hdhp.pdf, accessed September 6, 2014.

60. "2014 Employer Health Benefits Survey."
61. "2014 Employer Health Benefits Survey."

Chapter 4

THE DIFFERENCE BETWEEN HEALTH CARE AND HEALTH INSURANCE

"An older woman, I'd say she was in her sixties, walked into the clinic with a badly deformed arm. Although it didn't look like it hurt her, it was painful to see, and I've seen it all," said Mary Modigliani, a community clinic nurse. "She had an appointment with my doc, so I did the intake. Turns out she had broken her arm eight years ago but didn't have insurance and couldn't afford to pay for it to get fixed." Mary paused before saying, "Now that she was able on Obamacare, she wanted the doctor to see if he could fix it."

Mary explained what would happen next, "He'd have to pin it, and set it in a cast so it could heal properly. It would be very painful." The nurse shook her head," The problem is, it had been like that for so long, the muscles had atrophied. It would take a lot of physical therapy just to get it into a normal shape. I'm not sure it can even be done."

—Mary Modigliani, Community Clinic Nurse, Kaiser Permanente, Portland, Oregon.

The health insurance system in America needed reform as badly as health care itself. Prior to 2010, you could get health insurance only if you:

- Worked for a company that subsidized its cost as part of employee benefits.
- Could afford to pay for private insurance *and* had no preexisting conditions.
- Were very poor and qualified for Medicaid.
- Were 65 or older and qualified for Medicare.

If you didn't fall into one of those categories, you paid all medical expenses out of your own pocket. Since a typical doctor's visit costs anywhere from $100 to $300, not including tests and procedures, you probably just put it off as long as possible. A chronic condition, left untreated, could become a crisis. The average emergency room visit costs $1,265. If you ignored that suspicious mole or lump and developed cancer, the average cost of chemotherapy was $7,000, but could run as high as $30,000.

Like Mary's patient, you'd forgo treatment in some cases simply because you couldn't afford it. Otherwise, the hospital and treatment bills could wipe out your savings and force you to sell your home. After paying what you could, you'd have to declare bankruptcy and default on the rest. To make up for the loss, the hospital charged higher prices elsewhere, resulting in higher costs for everyone else, including health insurance companies.

To cover these expenses, the largest insurance companies gobbled up the smaller ones, dominating many markets. Prior to 2013, one or two companies in forty-five states controlled more than half the market for private (not employer-supplied) insurance. In fifteen states, a single company dominated the entire market. This problem was worse in large cities, where 71 percent of their insurance markets were dominated by one or two companies.

This removed the competitive pressure needed to keep premiums and other out-of-pocket costs low. It also raised expenses for doctors, especially those in small practices, because they lost their negotiating position when there weren't many insurance companies from which to choose.[1]

As a result, premiums more than doubled in the decade *before* the ACA was passed. The Kaiser Family Foundation found that the average premium for family plans (including the employer's share of costs) rose from $5,791 to $13,375 between 1999 and 2009. That's right, most people blame Obamacare for higher premiums, but cost escalation had been going on long before that.[2]

What Exactly *Is* Health Insurance?

Like insurance for your car, home, or apartment, health insurance is designed to protect your life savings from the devastating costs of a major incident. This could be anything from treating an accident, to a medical emergency (like a heart attack or hospitalization), or the expenses of a chronic health condition (like diabetes).

Unlike other types of insurance, however, health insurance is the gateway to life-saving treatments. If you total your car, and you don't have insurance to cover the costs, you can take the bus until you save up enough to buy a new one. If you break your leg, you can't splint it yourself until you save up enough to go to the doctor.

Therefore, health insurance has two goals: (1) protect your assets and (2) make sure you can get health care when you really need it. That's why most discussions about health-care reform in the United States are really about making insurance available to more people.

Health insurance is more complicated than auto or home insurance because it has four types of costs:

1. Premiums. Like any other kind of insurance, you pay a monthly premium just to have it. This gives insurance companies the regular cash flow they need to pay their day-to-day expenses and stay in business. How do health insurance companies decide on premium costs? They look at the pool of customers who are insured, how much they pay in premiums, and how many of them are older and/or sick. They raise premiums, if needed, to make sure they can pay the anticipated medical costs and still make a profit.

Premiums vary by state since insurance company costs are so variable. For example, if you have a high proportion of elderly people in your state, your premiums will be higher. Likewise, if the cost of living, especially health care, is higher in your state, that will put upward pressure on your premiums.

Just like auto or homeowners insurance, you pay premiums even if you never make a claim. If you're usually healthy, paying premiums year after year seems like a big waste of money. However, once you get hit with a massive hospital bill, and most of it is paid for by the insurance company, then the premium payments seem like a wise investment.

2. Co-payments. In addition to the premium, there is the co-payment for each visit. This is a fixed fee you pay each time you go to the doctor or the hospital, or buy a prescription medicine. A typical co-pay is $20 for a doctor visit, $50 for a hospital visit, and $10 to $40 for each prescription. For preventive care, your co-pay is zero thanks to the ACA.

3. Deductible. The deductible is the amount you must pay in qualified medical costs before the insurance "kicks in." Insurance companies added deductibles to plans to keep you from running to the doctor for every sniffle. They were worried that if health care were 100 percent free, their costs would skyrocket.

Deductibles can range anywhere from $500 a year (usually only available from company-sponsored plans) to $5,000 a year. They are annual, which means you start over January 1 of each year. Usually, the lower the deductible, the higher the premium, co-pay, or coinsurance. As health-care costs have grown, more people have opted for higher-deductible plans to keep their monthly premiums affordable.

4. Coinsurance. Once your deductible is met, you still have to pay the fourth cost, which is coinsurance. That's the percentage you pay versus the percent the insurance company pays for medical procedures. It's in addition to the co-payment. It's another way the insurance company makes sure you have "some skin in the game," sharing in the cost of health care so you don't use it frivolously.

Your deductible, co-payments, and coinsurance add up to your total out-of-pocket cost. Your out-of-pocket cost doesn't include the premiums and any costs that aren't covered, such as over-the-counter medicines. Thanks to the ACA, all companies now have an out-of-pocket maximum, after which you no longer pay coinsurance. In 2015, it's $6,600 for individuals and $13,200 for families. This amount rises each year to keep up with inflation. The out-of-pocket maximum protects your finances, so you don't have to pay hundreds of thousands of dollars for your part of the coinsurance. If insurance didn't protect you against this upside, it would be pretty useless.

You can choose a plan with the combination of payments that you want. For example, you might be willing to pay a higher monthly premium for a lower coinsurance percent and/or deductible. That would make sense if you have a chronic disease, like diabetes, and know you'll be in to see the doctor frequently. People who are usually healthy might want the lowest premium possible and a higher deductible. They are willing to take the chance of paying more for health care because they believe that chance is small.

Unfortunately, all this choice makes picking health-care insurance very complicated. You've got to be an odds-maker on your own health. How likely are you to get sick? What's your cash flow like? Do you have a lot of assets to protect? A step-by-step guide is in chapter 6 to help you with answering those questions and determining the right amount of insurance.

The Three Types of Health Insurance

There are three types of health insurance in the United States: government-provided, private group plans, and individual plans.

1. Government-provided plans can be at the federal, state, or local level—or even some combination of all three. The largest sub-category includes the federal plans designed to take care of specific groups of people: Medicare, Medicaid, and the Children's Health Insurance Program (CHIP).

Medicare is partially funded by contributions from payroll taxes, and so eligibility depends on whether you've contributed during your working life. However, these taxes aren't enough to cover the full cost, so part of it is paid out of the general fund. Medicaid and CHIP are also funded from the general fund and are awarded if you are below a certain income level. In addition, state governments help design, administer, and pay for Medicaid and CHIP for their residents.

Federal, state, and municipal governments also provide plans for their employees. This includes the Veterans Health Administration (VHA) and the Federal Employees Health Benefits (FEHB) Program.

2. Group plans are provided by employers, unions, and associations. Like most insurance, companies that offer group plans reduce their risk of paying out high health-care costs by averaging across a large number of mostly healthy people. That's because insurance companies are only profitable when more money is received in premiums than is paid out in claims. Averaging out the cost among a large group allows them to charge lower premiums to even chronically ill people. That's how group plans make health care affordable for their members.

The most common group plans are company-sponsored, covering sixty million people. In these plans, the company decides whether to offer benefits, the level of benefits, and amount of coverage. Employees simply choose whether to participate. They receive an insurance card that allows them to visit the doctors, hospitals, and other providers that are part of the plan. Employee premiums are usually subsidized by their employers. That's because companies can offer health insurance as an untaxed benefit. In a way, federal tax policies subsidize the employer-provided group insurance system.

Most companies work with major insurance companies such as UnitedHealth Group, Anthem, or Aetna. Large companies usually find it cheaper to self-insure, which simply means they pay for a portion of their employees' health costs themselves.

Not all companies are eligible to provide group plans. To be eligible, they must have at least two full-time owners, partners, or employees; must be a legal business entity; and must contribute to the plan.

Associations such as AARP, the Alliance for Affordable Services, the National Association for Female Executives, and various college alumni associations also offer group plans to its members. These are usually more expensive than employer-subsidized plans but cheaper than private plans.

3. Private health insurance covers the large group of people who don't qualify for government or group health insurance. These are typically the self-employed, those working for companies that don't offer insurance, part-time workers, those who lost their jobs, and people taking care of family members. Ironically, it also includes people who are too sick to work.

Before the ACA, about fifteen million people bought health insurance on their own. It was always the most expensive option, if you could get it at all. Insurance companies could deny you coverage if you had a preexisting disease or condition. For more, see chapter 5.

Why America Relies on Insurance to Pay for Health Care

Despite the cost of health care, hardly anyone had health insurance before World War II. The policies that existed only covered hospital room and board. After the war, inflation was out of control and the federal government froze prices and wages. As a result, companies couldn't give raises to get their best employees. Instead, they offered benefits, including health insurance.

In 1954, the IRS changed the tax laws regarding health insurance. The money that companies paid for their portion of your health insurance premiums was no longer included as part of taxable income. It became a tax break for the employee and the company. The Tax Policy Center estimated that the average benefit of the health insurance tax break is now about $800 for a household in the middle 20 percent of earners. The benefit is four times that, or $3,400, for people in the top 20 percent of the income range.[3]

However, that tax break eats into government revenue, increasing the deficit by $250 billion a year. It has the same impact as a government healthcare subsidy, except it only goes to those who are working for corporations that provide health insurance.[4]

The Impact of the High Cost of Health Insurance

The high cost of health care described in chapter 2 also increased the cost of health insurance. At first, businesses tried to absorb this increase. During the recession, they passed it along to their employees. At the same time, the recession forced many companies to hire part-time, temporary, and freelance employees instead of full-time workers—therefore saving the company costs of insurance and other benefits. Companies brought on contract labor only when they needed them and let them go when they didn't.

As a result, more and more people found they could not get employer-based health insurance. In 2000, more than two-thirds (69.7 percent) of employees got insurance from their job. By 2011, this had dropped to 59.5 percent. The CEA estimated that without healthcare reform the number of people without insurance would grow to 72 million by 2040.[5]

The rising cost of health insurance put small businesses and their employees at a disadvantage. Smaller companies stopped providing coverage because they simply couldn't afford it. Between 2000 and 2008, more than 90 percent of employers with twenty-five or more workers could afford to offer health benefits.

In 2000, 80 percent of those with ten to twenty-four workers offered these benefits, and even 57 percent of small (three to nine workers) companies could offer insurance. The ability to offer these benefits is absolutely necessary in order to hire the best workers.

By 2008, rising insurance costs had changed the landscape dramatically. While large companies continued to offer benefits, fewer of the smaller ones could afford to do so. Only 78 percent of the companies with ten to twenty-four workers offered insurance, while just 49 percent of those with three to nine workers did.

Larger companies can afford to self-insure. That means they just pay for the medical costs for their employees out of their own cash flow. This is cheaper for them than purchasing plans from an insurance company.

Even the large companies that purchase insurance for their employees pay less than small companies that are forced to buy small group plans. These plans cost 18 percent more than those for larger companies. This means more of the small companies' cash flow must go toward benefits instead of research, innovation, or building their business. This puts the small companies that do offer insurance at a competitive disadvantage.[6]

Why Health Insurance Costs So Much

The Supreme Court ruled that insurance is a business coupled with a public interest—not the healthiest combination. Much like a casino, the company is betting against you. In this case, the insurance company bets you won't get sick, while you're betting that you will. Government regulations protect you from this dangerous conflict of interest.

Regulations are also needed to protect you from poorly run insurance companies. These regulations help assess the insurance company's ability to make payments, assure that it's ethical, and try to provide fairness in coverage. They also oversee pricing, making sure companies don't lowball themselves out of business. Some companies may be really good at sales and customer service but poor at estimating their own costs, and therefore go bankrupt—leaving you holding the bag. Finally, regulations protect Americans against foreign firms that would just add another level of complexity.[7]

Health insurance companies must follow both federal and state regulations. Complying with this added layer of complexity adds to health insurance costs. Insurance plans are primarily regulated by the states, but some plans must also follow federal rules. For example, state laws cover benefits provided by local governments, churches, and individual private plans. They also cover all aspects of pricing, licensing, and claims. The federal laws regulate benefits provided by group plans offered by companies and unions.

1. The most important federal law is the Employee Retirement Income Security Act of 1974 (ERISA), which protects workers. It has five amendments that specifically cover health insurance benefits.
2. COBRA (Consolidated Omnibus Budget Reconciliation Act) requires group plans to offer coverage to workers for eighteen months if they lose their jobs.
3. HIPAA (the Health Insurance Portability and Accountability Act) forbids private insurers from denying coverage to people with preexisting conditions if they were covered by a group plan for the last eighteen months, or if they are applying for coverage in a group plan.
4. The Women's Health and Cancer Rights Act requires insurance companies to cover reconstructive surgery and complications after a mastectomy for breast cancer.
5. The Mental Health Parity Act requires plans that offer mental health benefits to make sure they are comparable to medical benefits.
6. The Newborns' and Mothers' Health Protection Act requires plans that offer maternity benefits to pay for at least a forty-eight hour stay, or ninety-six hours for cesarean sections.[8]

State regulations are usually managed by an insurance commission. The commission enforces regulations made by state legislatures and is funded by taxes on insurance premiums. As the insurance industry has grown in complexity, state regulations have not been able to keep up. In addition, the taxes are often diverted to other programs, leaving these commissions underfunded.

States establish regulations to make sure insurers can cover their obligations. However, they don't have the manpower to go into the field to inspect companies. Instead, they rely on reviews of annual financial statements. States are only supposed to license companies that have enough capital on hand to cover payments. However, many states set the requirements too low, licensing companies that aren't adequately funded. Most state commissions don't have the funds to prosecute those companies that do violate regulations. Many respond to consumer complaints by sending warning letters—but little else.

States are also responsible for regulating medical malpractice. The ACA provides additional funds for them to test malpractice reform. The ACA also extends federal malpractice protection to health-care providers in federal clinics.[9]

States set standards covering when and on what terms a state-licensed health insurer must accept an applicant. For example, most states mandate that coverage must be given to small employers that want to purchase coverage. States mandate the extent to which insurers can vary premiums based on health status, claims experience, and other factors. You can easily see how complicated it is for states to regulate health insurance.[10]

Why are states even involved? After the Civil War, many states realized they needed to supervise insurance within their boundaries. Insurance companies found their costs rising as they tried to create plans that adhered to the different laws for each state. To simplify their business, companies tried to get the Supreme Court to agree that insurance should be regulated only at the federal level. The Court disagreed, and further attempts to change the Constitution failed.[11]

As a result, the National Association of Insurance Commissioners (NAIC) now attempts to standardize state regulations over what is really a national, if not global, industry. Its members are state insurance commissioners, but it's funded by the insurance companies they are supposed to regulate. If companies don't like NAIC's regulations, they simply don't pay the fee. That results in a situation where the fox is guarding the hen house.[12]

Taxes on premiums, payments to NAIC, and staying on top of different state regulations increase the insurance companies' administration costs. This fosters the formation of monopoly power for the largest health insurance companies. That's because only the very large companies can adequately cover the cost of adhering to a variety of different state regulations. As a result, most states are dominated by only a few companies. The AMA found that 70 percent of the major metropolitan areas are "highly concentrated," meaning just a few insurance companies dominate these markets. In some states, only one company dominates the market. For example, a single insurer has 88 percent of Alabama's health insurance market.[13]

As a result, the five biggest health insurance companies—UnitedHealth Group, Anthem, Aetna, Humana, and Cigna service half of the insured population. That's more than one hundred million people. Anthem alone insures seventy million people. Never heard of WellPoint? It's the company that is behind the oldest health insurance plans in the country, those from Blue Cross and Blue Shield.[14]

In fact, a group of doctors and a group of patients have filed class action lawsuits against Blue Cross and Blue Shield insurers. They claim the licensed representatives have essentially formed a cartel that acts as a monopoly in setting prices for both what they pay doctors and what they charge patients. As of 2015, the cases were winding their way through the court system and could take years to settle. However, it would have a huge impact if the plaintiffs win, leading to a breakup of the big insurance companies.[15]

Between 1998 and 2010, more than four hundred mergers left Anthem and United-Health Group basically in control. Their revenue ($142 billion) was more than a third of the total market, while the top four earned $202 billion, nearly 75 percent of the market.

This consolidation gives these companies monopoly power. They can afford to hire more lobbyists at both the national and state legislatures. Between 2004 and 2010, they paid nearly $400 million to state legislatures. From 2008 to 2010, more than $1 billion overall had been spent to oppose reform.

The monopoly status of the largest health insurance companies enriches their shareholders and their managers. According to the Security and Exchanges Commission (SEC), their profits rose more than 400 percent between 2000 and 2008. The top executives were paid 468 times more than the average worker.[16]

In addition, companies have the power to tell doctors and hospitals which treatments they will cover and which ones they won't. This interferes with the doctor-patient relationship and might keep you from getting the right treatment.

Monopoly power gives insurance companies the ability to increase what they charge you. According to FamiliesUSA, premiums skyrocketed in many states way beyond those same states' wage increases. For example:

- California premiums skyrocketed 109 percent, while wages rose just 26 percent.
- New York premiums jumped 93 percent, while wages increased 14 percent.

- Texas premiums climbed 80 percent, while wages inched up just 11 percent.[17]

As mentioned earlier in this chapter, insurance companies have additional motives for raising your deductibles and co-payments. They are deliberately trying to discourage you from running to the doctor for every sniffle or to the emergency room for every chest pain. You're less likely to use your health care if you know it will cost you thousands because you haven't met the deductible. Even if you have, you'll think twice if it costs you hundreds of dollars in co-payments.

Insurance companies adopted this approach after a landmark 1974 study conducted by the RAND Corporation. It found that people who received free care used 40 percent more medical services than those who paid something out-of-pocket. For most people, the free care did not result in their improved health.

Insurers complained that free care especially led to overuse of emergency rooms. Those who had to pay something visited the emergency room 30 percent less than those with free care. If you're having a heart attack, you're calling 911 and going to the hospital— no matter what the cost. However, many decisions to go to the emergency room aren't so cut and dried.

If you break your arm, you'll go to the ER if you can afford it. If you can't, you'll wait until the next day and go to your doctor. Even chest pain can be ambiguous. Is it a heart attack or gas? The high cost of the emergency room means many people will delay receiving care until it's too late. The RAND study found that people who had to pay even a portion of ER costs were 23 percent less likely to go *even when they really needed it*. Therefore, even though deductibles do cut costs for insurance companies, this may not be in the best interest of patients.[18]

Another reason health insurance costs increased so much was because insurance companies charged an extra $1,000 a year in premiums per family (on average) to compensate them for people who receive services but don't have insurance. How is that possible? Hospitals are required by law to treat everyone who walks through the emergency room door. If that person doesn't pay, the hospital must make up the cost by charging everyone else a little more. Those costs are borne by health insurance companies. For them to remain profitable, they've got to raise premiums for everyone else.[19]

Are Health Insurance Companies Evil?

Many people believe insurance companies are evil, crooks, or even run by the Mafia. They misconstrue corporate motives, forgetting that insurance companies are in business to make a profit. *Wall Street Journal* columnist Jonathan Kellerman explains why people feel this way. He says that all middlemen that come between a buyer and seller will raise the price. Most do so while providing additional benefits, such as expertise, advertising, or transportation. Others use fear to muscle their way into the provider-consumer relationship.

Kellerman compares health insurance to the Mafia since both provide nothing other than "protection." He adds that, unlike the Mafia, insurance companies first blend themselves into the legitimate system. Then, they increase their profit by changing the rules about what they will and won't cover. This harms the people they are allegedly protecting by reducing service.

Any kind of protection is about betting against negative consequences. The insurance business is unique because it only makes money when its service is *not* being provided. Companies "place their bets" by using actuarial tables to determine the risk. They use these tables to set what they should charge to cover that risk. This additional knowledge gives these companies an unfair advantage. They know the likelihood you will need health care, based on your age, gender, and prior history. You don't have the same access to these detailed statistics. They can use this data to lower their costs by denying authorization of services, increasing co-payments, and lowering payments to doctors.[20]

Chapter 4: References

1. "AMA Analysis Lists States Where One Private Health Insurer Rules," American Medical Association, November 7, 2013. http://www.ama-assn.org/ama/pub/news/news/2013/2013-11-07-study-anticompetitive-market-conditions.page, accessed October 11, 2014.

2. "Employer Health Benefits," Kaiser Family Foundation, 20009. http://kaiserfamilyfoundation.files.wordpress.com/2013/04/7936.pdf, accessed November 1, 2014.

3. Pat Regnier, "The Hidden Health Care Subsidy for the Rich," *Money*, August 5, 2014. http://time.com/money/3080674/obamacare-subsidy-affluent-tax-break/, accessed August 31, 2014.

4. Ezekiel J. Emanuel, "Inside the Making of Obamacare," *Wall Street Journal*, March 7, 2014. http://online.wsj.com/news/articles/SB10001424052702303824204579421553914382752, accessed October 11, 2014.

5. "Number of Americans Obtaining Health Insurance Through an Employer Declines Steadily Since 2000," Robert J. Woods Foundation, April 11, 2013. http://www.rwjf.org/en/library/articles-and-news/2013/04/number-of-americans-obtaining-health-insurance-through-an-employ.html, accessed October 7, 2014.

6. Commonwealth Fund, "How Will Comprehensive Reform Improve Health Care for Americans?" October 2009. http://www.commonwealthfund.org/~/media/Files/Publications/Other/2009/Sep/CF%20Insert%20FINAL.pdf, accessed October 6, 2014.

7. Susan Randall, "Insurance Regulation in the United States," Florida State University College of Law, 1999, p. 627, 2014. http://www.law.fsu.edu/journals/lawreview/downloads/263/rand.pdf, accessed August 31, 2014.

8. "ERISA," Department of Labor. http://www.dol.gov/dol/topic/health-plans/erisa.htm, accessed October 9, 2014.

9. Emanuel, "Inside the Making."

10. "How Health Insurance Works," Health Care Services Corporation. http://www.hcsc.com/how_insurance_works.html, accessed October 8, 2014.

11. Randall, "Insurance Regulation," p. 631.

12. Randall, "Insurance Regulation," p. 640.

13. "New AMA Study Find Anticompetitive Market Conditions Are Common Across Managed Care Plans," American Medical Association, November 28, 2012. http://www.ama-assn.org/ama/pub/news/news/2012-11-28-study-finds-anticompetitive-market-conditions-common.page, accessed October 9, 2014.

14. Amanda Baltazar, "The Big Five: Health Insurance Companies," About.com. http://pharmacy.about.com/od/Insurance/a/The-Big-Five-Health-Insurance-Companies.htm, accessed October 9, 2014.

15. Anna Wilde Mathews, "Antitrust Suites Target Blue Cross," *Wall Street Journal*, May 28, 2015.

16. Don Monkerud, "The Health Insurance Monopoly," Counterpunch.org, January 14, 2010. http://www.counterpunch.org/2010/01/14/the-health-insurance-monopoly/, accessed October 9, 2014.

17. Monkerud, "The Health Insurance Monopoly."

18. Harold Pollack, "Lessons from an Emergency Room Nightmare," *The American Prospect*, December 17, 2008. http://www.alternet.org/story/113091/lessons_from_an_emergency_room_nightmare, accessed November 1, 2014.

19. Seung Min Kim, "Study: Insured Pay Hidden Cost," *USA Today*, May 29, 2009. http://usatoday30.usatoday.com/money/industries/insurance/2009-05-28-hiddentax_N.htm, October 7, 2014.

20. Jonathan Kellerman, "The Health Insurance Mafia," *Wall Street Journal*, April 14, 2008. http://online.wsj.com/articles/SB120813453964211685, accessed October 8, 2014.

Chapter 5

THE ACA REFORMS HEALTH INSURANCE

You probably think that Obamacare mainly raises your taxes and health-care insurance premiums so the poor can get free health care, right? That's what most people think, and it's because the media and critics have portrayed it that way. In fact, the ACA does raise taxes and it does help millions of poor families get Medicaid.

More importantly, the ACA standardizes all health insurance plans, doing away with a lot of hidden clauses that insurance companies previously used to prevent you from getting many of the benefits you probably thought you were getting.

The Ten Essential Benefits

Now, all plans must provide some level of coverage in each of these ten essential benefit categories:

1. **Preventive and wellness visits, such as well-woman visits, domestic violence screening, and chronic disease management.** The ACA requires insurance companies, and Medicare, to pay 100 percent of these costs.
2. **Lab tests.** Plans must cover 100 percent of preventive tests.
3. **Maternity and newborn care.** This is considered preventive care and is therefore 100 percent covered.
4. **Pediatric care.** The ACA requires plans to cover dental and vision care for children.
5. **Prescription drugs.** Most plans offered some kind of drug coverage at an extra cost. The ACA now requires plans to include coverage of at least one drug in every category in the US Pharmacopeia. Whatever you pay out-of-pocket for drugs will also count toward your deductible, which wasn't true before for all plans.
6. **Mental and behavioral health treatment.** All plans must include treatment for alcohol, drug, and other substance abuse and addiction.

7. **Services and devices to help people with injuries, disabilities, or chronic conditions.** Most plans cover services and equipment to help you recover from temporary injuries, like a broken leg. The ACA requires plans to cover goods and services to help you maintain a standard of living if you contract a chronic disease, like multiple sclerosis.

8. **Emergency room.** Most plans already covered emergency room treatment. However, they can no longer charge extra for an out-of-network visit, or require pre-authorization, thanks to the ACA.

9. **Hospitalization.** Most plans covered this, but they had annual and lifetime limits. The ACA prohibits these limits.

10. **Outpatient care, such as doctor visits.** The ACA requires plans to provide a sufficiently large network size to give patients some choice in treatment.[1]

Your Benefit Checklist

There's a laundry list of other benefits the ACA provides that are designed to make health insurance more convenient, affordable, and straightforward. Below is a checklist. How many did you know you were now receiving? How many did you know came from the ACA?

- Plans can't make you wait more than ninety days before coverage starts.
- Your out-of-pocket costs can't exceed $6,600 for an individual plan or $13,200 for a family plan (2015 limit).
- Small market plans must cover the ten essential health benefits.
- Plans can't drop you because you've entered a clinical trial for cancer or other life-threatening disease.
- Plans must cover 100 percent of the cost (that means no co-pays) for preventive services such as mammograms and colonoscopies.
- You can appeal claim rejections or other health insurance decisions through your state regulator.
- The exchanges allow you to compare, price, and purchase health insurance online.
- You can also compare doctors, hospitals, and other providers in your area.

- In addition to signing up at the online exchanges, you can get free, local, face-to-face, or telephone help in applying for insurance.
- Your children can stay on your plan until they turn twenty-six.
- Employers must give mothers time from work and a private room to nurse their babies or express milk.
- Your employer must give you a uniform summary of benefits and coverage and a sixty-day advance notice if anything changes in your coverage.
- Insurance companies for large employer plans must spend at least 85 percent of all premium dollars on health-care service benefits, not administration or advertising. This drops to 80 percent for plans sold to individuals and small employers. If insurance companies do not meet these goals, they must send rebates back to consumers. You might have already received your rebate and not known it was because of Obamacare.
- If you have Medicare Part D, the "donut hole" that you have to pay on your drug plan will be eliminated by 2020. You also receive free wellness exams and preventive tests.
- Small businesses can get a tax credit worth up to 50 percent of their contribution to their employees' health insurance if purchased on the SHOP exchange. Nonprofits receive a 35 percent credit. Find out how at www.healthcare.gov/small-businesses/provide-shop-coverage/small-business-tax-credits/ or www.healthcare.gov/small-businesses/provide-shop-coverage/choose-shop-insurance/.
- If you're a doctor, the ACA requires states to make sure the Medicaid payments you receive are no lower than payment rates for Medicare.

The ACA also provides additional benefits:

- Funds scholarships and loans to double the number of health-care providers in five years.
- Cuts down on fraudulent doctor/supplier relationships. The ACA invests new resources and requires new screening procedures for health-care providers to reduce fraud and waste in Medicare, Medicaid, and CHIP.[2]
- Requires background checks of all nursing home staff to protect elders from abuse.
- Provides $250 million to states to better regulate excessive insurance rate hikes.

- Established the CMS Innovation Center, as mentioned in chapter 3, to create a national strategy to improve health care and lower costs.
- Created the Independent Payment Advisory Board to recommend ways to reduce costs while improving the quality of care.
- Charged the National Prevention Council to coordinate all federal health efforts to reduce drug abuse.
- Added $15 billion to the Prevention and Public Health Fund to invest in proven public health programs, from smoking cessation to combating obesity.
- Added funding to attract doctors to medically underserved communities in rural areas.
- Created the Community First Choice Option to encourage states to offer home- and community-based services to disabled individuals through Medicaid. This lowers costs by keeping them out of nursing homes.

These are all great benefits and protections. However, many insurance companies dropped their plans because it was too expensive for them to comply. This is the major reason millions of people lost their insurance coverage. People accused President Obama of lying when he said, "You can keep your insurance. Period." It's also the reason that many people think the cost of insurance is higher under Obamacare. Most don't realize it's because they are getting more coverage than in their old plans.

What most people didn't realize, until it was too late, was that their old plans didn't really protect them when they needed it. For example, did you know that your insurance plan could refuse payment for your treatment if it found any errors on your application? That it could drop you after an expensive procedure? That, even if it did pay for your treatment and didn't drop you, it would probably raise your premiums the following year?

The next three sections of chapter 5 go into detail about three more benefits that are so important they deserve detailed explanations. The first big benefit is a ruling that prevents insurance companies from denying you a policy because you have, or get, a disease. This is known as a preexisting condition, and it kept millions from getting coverage.

The second benefit that helps people regardless of income is the elimination of annual and lifetime limits. This is particularly important for those with chronic conditions, such as hemophiliacs and many premature babies.

The third is the ACA's emphasis on preventive care, which is now 100 percent covered by insurance. It funds community health centers to treat those who would otherwise use expensive emergency rooms as a primary care facility. It also allows employer-sponsored health plans to give a discount to employees who meet specific standards in criteria such as blood pressure, glucose, or cholesterol—key indicators of preventable chronic disease.

Preexisting Conditions: Why Fifty Million People Couldn't Get Insured

Rose Carey and her husband, Mike, were on their way to brunch when they saw a yard sale that had a pasta-maker on display. After snatching it up, Mike asked the owner of the yard sale, "Are you moving?" The woman replied, "No. I'm trying to raise money for my operation. I lost my job when I was sick last year and now don't have insurance to cover it. I'm too sick to work full-time, and every time I apply for private insurance . . ." she hesitated. "Well, once the companies see the diagnosis of 'brain tumor,' I always get rejected. At this point, unless I get married or find a full-time job that allows part-time work, I'm on my own. I've applied for Medicaid, but I don't know if I'll get it in time."

Months later, Rose and Mike drove by the corner again on their way to brunch and noticed two small boys playing in the yard. They were tempted to stop and find out what happened to the woman . . . but by then, they had driven past.

This story was all too common in pre-ACA America. There were fifty million people who, like the lady having the yard sale, had a serious condition that would have prevented them from getting private health insurance. Of those, four million were children.

However, you didn't have to have brain cancer to be refused health insurance. Many were denied due to common diseases, like asthma, arthritis, and even high blood pressure (more on those later in this chapter). Combined, the number of people with preexisting conditions nearly tripled to 129 million, with seventeen million under the age of 18. That's half of the population not on Medicare.

The reason you didn't hear more about it is that eighty-two million of those with pre-existing conditions were in group plans. If you're one of those people, you haven't had to worry about being denied insurance due to your preexisting condition. That's thanks to HIPAA, previously mentioned in chapter 4.

HIPAA restricted the use of preexisting condition clauses for group plans. It allowed these plans to cover you for everything but the preexisting condition. It set a "look-back" period—if you were symptom-free during that time, then they had to cover the preexisting condition. If you had continuous insurance coverage, then the new plan had to cover you. Unfortunately, these HIPAA requirements did not apply to private plans.

The reason that group plans were able to cover those with preexisting conditions was because their groups had enough healthy people in them to pay for the sick people. If that sounds unfair to the healthy people, remember that's how insurance works. All the people who never have accidents pay premiums each month to cover the insurance company's payments to those who do.

The situation for those without company plans was very different. Nearly half (47 percent) of those with preexisting conditions who sought private insurance were flat out refused coverage, charged a higher premium, or had their condition excluded because of it.

Another 26 percent were denied coverage for what the insurance company considered a preexisting condition even though they were healthy. For example, if you've ever had chronic back pain, some companies denied you coverage for that. Others denied you coverage for going to the chiropractor to treat the back pain. It was very frustrating to go through the lengthy application process, submit paper records from all your doctors, and then months later be denied coverage for "chronic back problems," even though records showed you were taking preventive measures to alleviate those problems. If you've never had to get private health insurance on your own, you'd be surprised at how difficult it was.[3]

It's easy to see why an insurance company wouldn't want the risk of someone with cancer, heart disease, or diabetes. That's like a car insurance company accepting someone with eleven DUIs.

But, if you're relatively healthy, you'd expect them to welcome you with open arms. In all likelihood, you'd be paying premiums year after year without one trip to the emergency room. The insurance companies didn't see it that way, because they didn't have to. Each company made up its own definition of a preexisting condition because there were no laws governing them.

What Qualified as a Preexisting Condition?

Insurance companies considered any health condition that was diagnosed or treated by a health-care provider during the previous twelve months as a preexisting condition. This included symptoms that caused "an ordinarily prudent person to seek diagnosis or treatment," even if the doctor said you were healthy. If companies didn't deny you coverage outright, they might only provide coverage for everything but the condition. Once a year went by without a recurrence of the condition, then they would fully cover you.

Below are examples of some of the most prevalent preexisting conditions, with their incidences if available.

AIDS—There are 1.2 million people in the United States who are HIV-positive. The Centers for Disease Control and Prevention (CDC) adds that one in seven are completely unaware they even have it.

Alzheimer's—Over five million people in the United States have Alzheimer's, the most common form of dementia, according to the CDC.

Alcoholism—There are 17.6 million people who suffer from alcohol abuse or dependence. An additional seven million children live in a household where a parent is dependent on alcohol. More than half of all adults have a family history of alcoholism. The CDC reports that thirty-eight million people binge drink at least four times a month. Binge drinking is eight drinks per binge. Excessive alcohol use is involved in 10 percent of deaths among working-age adults.[4]

Cancer—Each year, more than 1.6 million people are diagnosed with cancer. That's in addition to the 14.5 million cancer survivors.[5]

Diabetes—According to the CDC, 20.9 million people in the United States have diabetes.

Drug abuse—Twenty million people, or 8 percent of the population age twelve and older, used an illegal drug in the past thirty days. There are forty-eight million people who use prescription drugs such as painkillers, sedatives, and stimulants for nonmedical reasons. That's twenty percent of the population.[6]

Fatty liver disease—This disease occurs when more than 5 to 10 percent of your liver is made up of fat cells. Over time, it can lead to cirrhosis and is one of the most common causes of liver disease. Nearly all of the twenty million people who abuse alcohol either have liver disease or will get it. In addition, there's another 20 percent of the population who have non-alcoholic fatty liver. It can come from diabetes, obesity, high cholesterol, hepatitis, or even malnutrition.[7]

Heart attack—Around 735,000 people have a heart attack each year. Nearly half receive no warning. That's in addition to the eight million people who have had a heart attack, and survived.[8]

Inflammatory bowel/Crohn's disease—From 1 to 1.3 million people suffer from either Crohn's or ulcerative colitis.[9]

Pacemakers—In 2009, pacemakers were put into 188,700 people.[10]

Kidney failure—Each year, more than 113,000 people start treatment for kidney failure. More than twenty million people may have chronic kidney disease. However, one-third of those with diabetes and 20 percent of those with high blood pressure also have some level of kidney disease.[11]

Rheumatoid arthritis—1.5 million Americans have the disease. This is not to be confused with the 26.9 million people with osteoarthritis.[12]

Stroke—About eight hundred thousand Americans have a stroke each year. Nearly 130,000 die from it.[13]

Although you can understand why an insurance company would reject anyone with these diseases, when you look at the numbers, you can also see why so many millions of people could not get insurance at all.

To make matters worse, insurance companies also considered the following situations that were not actually diseases to be preexisting conditions.

Intellectual disability—There are at least 4.6 million Americans with an IQ (Intelligence Quotient) that's measured at seventy or below. Many more are misdiagnosed as someone with a learning disability, behavior disorder, or autism.[14]

Mental health counseling—Anyone who was in counseling was automatically denied. Insurance companies would only consider people who were finished with counseling for at least six months, and many would still be denied depending on the reason for counseling. For example, marriage counseling was fine, but drug counseling was not.

Weight—If your Body Mass Index (BMI) was above the normal range, you were charged 25 percent extra. However, if your BMI was more than a maximum set by the insurance company, you were denied.

Isn't this discrimination? Not according to the insurance companies. That's because obesity leads to the major causes of preventable death: heart disease, stroke, diabetes, and even some types of cancer. The medical costs for an obese person are $1,429 higher each year than for someone of normal weight.[15]

Pregnancy—There were more than 6.5 million pregnancies in 2008 (latest data). If you were pregnant when you applied for health insurance, you'd be denied. You'd usually have to wait a year after getting the insurance before you became pregnant. Otherwise, the plan didn't have to offer maternity benefits. [16]

Even if you weren't sick and didn't have a preexisting condition listed above, but simply took preventive care, it could count against you. For example, say you mentioned to your doctor during your annual physical exam that you had chest pains while running a few months ago. He ordered you to take a stress test, and the results were clear. From that, he concluded your pains were due to anxiety. That would count as a preexisting heart condition, preventing you from getting private health insurance should you apply for it.

Even minor conditions, such as hay fever, a previous surgery, or an injury from an accident, often counted as a preexisting condition. As you can see, this pretty much included everyone.

And forget about lying, or even forgetting something, on an application. If the company found an inconsistency in your application once you applied for a claim, it could deny the claim or even cancel your policy. This meant that, before applying for insurance, you'd have to get a copy of your medical records and copy it word-for-word into your insurance application to make sure you remembered everything.

Who Benefits from the ACA's Coverage of Preexisting Conditions?

Darcy Liggett was a successful sales rep at Boeing. Her husband, Bob, owned his own natural herb supplement business, which he used to treat his chronic Crohn's disease. Darcy's insurance paid for his hospitalizations and his surgeries. She sometimes joked that he married her for her insurance since his preexisting condition prevented him from getting a private plan on his own.

Although Darcy did well at her job, the constant travel was making her miserable. The couple had saved enough for them to retire when Bob turned fifty-five, but now Darcy realized that dream was impossible. She had to keep working until he turned sixty-five and qualified for Medicare.

In 2010, the ACA banned insurance companies from denying coverage to children with preexisting conditions. The ban went into effect for adults in 2014. As a result, your insurance company can no longer deny you coverage because you are already sick.[17]

Similarly, insurance companies can't withhold coverage once you become sick, especially if it's because of a preexisting condition. They also can't charge you extra because of your preexisting condition.

Those with Preexisting Conditions

If you are one of the millions with a preexisting condition, you no longer have to worry whether you can afford to pay for your health care. You don't have to stay with a job you can't stand because of the benefits.

Those Who Have Family Members with Preexisting Conditions

Like Darcy, you could be affected by a family member's preexisting condition even if you didn't have one yourself. If your family member couldn't get insurance, they might rely on you for coverage. If your employer provided health insurance, you'd be stuck at that job just for the benefits. If not, you'd have to find a job that did provide that insurance. Your income and career would be centered around insurance, not the best use of your skills, what you enjoyed, or what provided the highest salary.

Society-at-Large

If you're one of the few who has never been touched by a preexisting condition, you'll still benefit from this aspect of Obamacare. That's because those who had no health insurance and were forced to use the emergency room as a primary care physician cost the entire health system the most.

A study done in Camden, New Jersey, showed that just 1 percent of its 79,000 residents ran up 30 percent of the City's hospital emergency room costs. These 386 so-called super-users averaged thirteen emergency room visits each in 2011. That's 5,000 trips in total. Most of them "shop hospitals" to find the best care, treating emergency room staff as their own personal family doctors.

If they can be treated for their illnesses at a low-cost urgent care or doctor's office, it will reduce health-care expenses for everyone dramatically. For example, a fifty-five-year-old man with nine chronic preexisting conditions visited the ER nine times in one year. His treatment cost $312,000, of which Medicare and Medicaid paid $59,000. The rest was the hospital's loss that was transmitted as higher prices to everyone else, including insurance companies.

He was assigned a coordinated care manager at Camden Coalition, which managed his home care, transport, meals, crutches, wheelchair, and dialysis. Once his preexisting conditions were treated, he didn't need to visit the emergency room for the next six months—lowering costs for everyone. [18]

Pros and Cons

Allowing people with chronic, preexisting conditions to get insurance should lower health-care costs over the long run. As mentioned previously, they'll be able to get preventive care that keeps them out of the emergency room.

However, health insurance companies warn that allowing all those people with preexisting conditions to suddenly run to the doctor will cost them more money than anyone realizes. As a result, companies will have to either raise premiums or cut earnings forecasts. The first solution will make policyholders and voters unhappy, while the second solution will make stockholders and industry associations unhappy. Both will make politicians unhappy, one of the reasons why a new president may yet find a way to repeal Obamacare after 2016.

Ways Insurance Companies Get Around the Preexisting Condition Rules

Since insurance companies are worried about the costs of paying for those with preexisting conditions, some have come up with ways to legally get around the ACA rules.

For example, some are putting the drugs needed by high-cost patients, like those with AIDS, on a more expensive tier. Three insurers in Florida—CoventryOne, Cigna, and Preferred Medical—also require HIV/AIDS patients to pay 40 percent of the costs of these drugs. That can run as much as $1,000 a month, depending on the specific drug.

The ACA does restrict out-of-pocket costs to $6,350 a year, but HIV/AIDS patients will easily spend that amount in six months. These companies are trying to drive the high-cost patients to other plans, such as those licensed by Blue Cross and Blue Shield that charge no more than $70 per drug. In Louisiana, some insurance companies refuse to accept third-party payments for organizations that treat HIV/AIDS patients.

This doesn't just happen to HIV/AIDS patients. Drugs to treat multiple sclerosis and some forms of cancer are also placed on the most expensive cost-sharing tier. A recent Avalere Health study found the more than 60 percent of 123 mid-level companies on the health exchange did just that.[19]

Insurance companies can also choose not to list certain name-brand drugs at all. The list of drugs they cover is called a formulary. The states legislate the types of drugs that must be on this list. Insurance companies must comply with the states' benchmarks.

Most companies will choose a cheaper generic rather than a name-brand drug. If your doctor requires you to have the name-brand drug, and your insurance company doesn't cover it, the ACA has an appeals process.

If you buy a drug that's not on the formulary, it won't count against your deductible or the out-of-pocket limit. Therefore, it's a good idea to check the insurance company's formulary before you sign up.[20]

Annual and Lifetime Limits: Their Elimination Saves You Money

Little Chloe Harper had her first open-heart surgery when she was fifteen months old. Before her first birthday, she was halfway to the annual limit that health insurance plans were allowed to impose. Thanks to the ACA, her mother Amber can now afford the care Chloe needs. That's because all plans issued since September 23, 2010, have no annual limits.

Annual and lifetime limits allowed insurance companies to really only pay a fixed portion of your health bill—the amount greater than your deductible but less than the limit. Before the ACA, your insurance plans probably had a limit, usually $1 million, on how much insurance you could use that year. The lifetime limit was typically from $1 million to $2.5 million.

That meant that, after you paid the deductible, the plan would pay up to that point each year of their share. You still had to pay your coinsurance, your co-payment, and your premiums. Once the plan hit the limit, you had to pay 100 percent of the rest.

Depending on your deductible, it could mean they wouldn't cover a broken leg ($2,500) because that was less than a typical deductible. They also wouldn't cover the amount beyond the $1 million limit. That could be as much as $200,000 for either an intestinal or heart-lung transplant, because those cost around $1.2 million each.

Other common, expensive procedures are below the $1 million cut-off themselves, but could have easily pushed you beyond the annual limit if you had any other illnesses or procedures that year. These include:

- Heart transplant—$997,700
- Bone marrow transplant—from $300,400 to $676,800, depending on whether surgery is needed
- Lung transplant—$561,200 for one, $797,200 for both
- Liver transplant—$577,100
- Open-heart surgery—$324,000
- Pancreas transplant—$289,400
- Kidney transplant—$262,900
- Tracheostomy—$205,000[21]

Doctors can now keep treating children like Chloe, who were more likely to reach the annual cap before they were well. Why were children particularly vulnerable to annual caps? Advances in medical care for premature infants allow them to survive at younger and younger ages. Unfortunately, it also means they require more extensive surgery to correct organs that haven't quite developed yet. These costs can go on for years if one surgery isn't enough.

Lifetime Limits Meant the Chronically Ill Lost Coverage

In addition to an annual limit, your plan probably had a limit on how much it would cover in your lifetime. Typically, this lifetime limit was between $1 and $2.5 million. You probably never knew it because fortunately you never hit it. However, it was a ticking time bomb for the 105 million people who had plans with a lifetime limit, including nearly twenty-eight million children.

You had a better-than-even chance of being one of the ninety-one million whose company plans had a lifetime limit. More than half (59 percent) of insured people were on those plans in 2009, according to the Kaiser Family Foundation Benefits Survey.

The odds were much worse for those who bought a private plan. Nearly all (89 percent) of them had plans with a lifetime limit.[22]

However, it was a real and painful reality for the twenty-five thousand who lost their insurance because they exceeded the lifetime limit, according to a PricewaterhouseCoopers study in 2009. Without the ACA, that number would have increased to 300,000 people by 2019.

Why the tremendous increase in just ten years? Most companies hadn't raised the limit in decades. While the cost of health care rose each year, the limit didn't. Each year, more and more people hit the limit for that simple reason.[23]

How easy was it to rack up enough expenses to reach the limit? Too easy, if your baby was born extremely prematurely, if someone on your plan needed an organ transplant, or if someone came down with a blood infection that led to system failure requiring multiple hospitalizations.

For example, one out of every nine babies are born prematurely (at least three weeks early). These tiny infants are more likely to have intellectual disabilities, cerebral palsy, or deafness.[24]

Imagine if, during your next pregnancy, you wake up in the middle of the night with contractions—and you are seventeen weeks early! Your baby is born, weighing only one or two pounds, and is rushed into a neonatal intensive care unit, receiving round-the-clock care.

You spend the next three months watching your baby as he's hooked up to life support, trying to grow while receiving drugs and surgeries to correct common preemie complications. These include bleeding in the brain, scarring in the lungs, or intestinal problems. The last thing you want to do is worry about how to pay the bill once the insurance runs out! Especially if you've been paying premiums all your life.

In countries with socialized medicine, like the Netherlands, you wouldn't have to worry about it. That's because they don't try to save those babies. Doctors there don't provide active, intensive treatment for babies delivered younger than twenty-six weeks. Most of those babies don't survive and those that do usually have severe disabilities.

However, as Dr. Phil Kibort, MD, chief medical officer at Children's Hospitals and Clinics of Minnesota, said, "In the United States, our society has said we want to save these babies." This does increase health-care costs for society, but he adds, "The dilemma is, if that was your baby, what would you want me to do?"[25]

Most of us would probably say we are proud to live in a society where the government doesn't decide who gets to live and who gets to die. However, think of it this way. The health insurance system before the ACA did, through default, decide that those who lost the genetic lottery and couldn't afford to spend millions on health care were more likely to die. By leaving it up to the private insurance market, the government made that decision in absentia.[26]

It's too easy to exceed the lifetime limit if your baby has hemophilia (400 born each year), a congenital defect, or a metabolic disease like Tay-Sachs or Gaucher disease. Or your child could get cancer, the leading cause of disease-related death in children. The National Cancer Institute says that 15,780 children (younger than 19 years) were diagnosed with some form of cancer in 2014. Sadly, nearly 2,000 would die from it.[27]

Imagine being stuck in the impossible situation of finding hundreds of thousands of dollars to keep your child alive after the insurance ran out. That's because a lifetime limit meant that the insurance company would cut you off after your expense reached a certain amount. That's it—no more insurance from that company for the rest of your (or your child's) life. The preexisting condition clause meant you would be highly unlikely to find another private plan. Therefore, you'd have to change jobs to find a group plan that would take you.

There are 20,000 hemophiliacs in the United States today. Although most had a family history of the disease, one-third had no idea. That's because sometimes a gene spontaneously mutates.

People with chronic illnesses, like hemophilia, had to try to estimate when their lifetime limit would be exceeded so they could prepare to get a different insurance plan or find more money.

Ted Barnes, a teenage boy with hemophilia, needed three treatments a week so his blood would clot normally. Otherwise, even a simple paper cut could have killed him. At an annual cost of $316,000 a year, the limit would be reached in just six years. To make things worse, 80 to 90 percent of hemophiliacs contracted HIV and/or Hepatitis C due to contamination of the nation's blood supply in the 1980s.[28]

Annual Limits Meant You Could Only Have One Serious Illness a Year

Nicole Mitchell, an active twenty-six-year-old mother of two boys, fell while hiking with her family in 2009 and cut her knee. When she got home, she put some alcohol and a bandage on it and started grilling hot dogs.

A week later she noticed it was infected, with a hard knot under it. That weekend, she woke up with so much pain she thought someone had plunged a hot knife into her knee. She went to the urgent care clinic the next morning. To her surprise, they immediately rushed her to the hospital.

Sure enough, she had MRSA. She was admitted and put on a wide-spectrum intravenous antibiotic while they cultured the bacteria that had infected her. By the time they found the drug that would work, the infection had spread to her bloodstream. She was on dialysis and ventilators, and her medication cost $1,600 a dose.

While her family prayed for her recovery, her husband Dan realized the bills would exceed the $1 million annual limit imposed by his insurance. They'd have to take out a second mortgage on their house, deplete the boys' college fund, and potentially wipe out their 401(k).

Fortunately, Nicole recovered in time and is back to hiking again. But Dan was so shaken, and they came so close to the lifetime limit, he changed jobs to a company that offered health insurance with no limit—even though it meant a cut in pay.

Dan didn't realize how lucky he was, even if he had stayed with the old company. If he had worked for himself and gotten private insurance, the insurance company would have canceled his plan. And, thanks to the prohibitions individual insurers had against preexisting conditions, he'd have a hard time finding a new one.

If you think that's rare, you're behind the times. Since 2000, the hospitalization rate for septicemia or sepsis (the medical term for what happened to Nicole) has doubled. The number of cases has increased from 621,000 to 1.141 million in 2008.[29]

If this had happened to you, and your insurance was from your place of employment, you'd have to sign up with another plan once you reached the annual limit. If your company didn't offer another plan, you'd have to switch jobs to get a different provider. To cope, many people found jobs just so they could get on unlimited group plans. Others got married or stayed married for the same reasons.

What then? Many were able to convince their employers to raise the limit. Once that was hit, they could try to find an expensive plan that would cover their disease. Some could switch to their spouse's plan. Others put off needed surgeries to delay reaching the limit.[30]

Eventually, those with chronic illnesses were forced to spend all their money until they went bankrupt. That's one reason health-care costs are the number one cause of bankruptcy.[31]

Once all other avenues were exhausted and they were penniless, they qualified for Medicaid. In other words, the federal government picked up the slack left by insurance companies.

How much? The 2009 PricewaterhouseCoopers study found that Medicaid programs would save $1 billion a year if lifetime limits were raised to at least $10 million. Companies were willing to do this under Obamacare because they would receive millions of new customers thanks to the mandate. More on this in chapter 8.[32]

Warning: Some Plans Still Have Annual and Lifetime Limits

Some private insurance plans may still have annual and lifetime limits. Check the date that you received your plan. If you received it before January 1, 2014, it may still include these limits:

- Plans starting before September 23, 2010, were grandfathered in and may retain annual limits.
- Plans starting between September 23, 2010, and September 22, 2011, can't have an annual limit less than $750,000.
- Plans starting on or after September 23, 2011, can't have an annual limit less than $1.25 million.

- Plans issued between September 23, 2012, and January 1, 2014, can't have an annual limit less than $2 million.

In addition, plans can put annual and lifetime limits on spending for health-care services that are not included as one of the ten essential benefits. Plans can also limit the number of days treatment is received, number of visits, or number of prescriptions. Other plans may have special circumstances.[33]

Double-check all plans for these contingencies, especially if you bought it outside of the exchange. If your plan does have an annual or lifetime limit, find a new one. There's no point in having insurance that doesn't protect your home and assets from truly expensive medical procedures.

Prevention: A (Not So) New and Simple Plan for Cutting Health Costs

Tom Fielding first noticed the suspicious mole on his arm in 2013. As a self-employed hairdresser, he had never been able to afford private health insurance and knew he'd have trouble getting any coverage if it were diagnosed as cancer. He was one of the first to sign up for Obamacare on the marketplace.

The biopsy showed it was cancer. Thanks to the ACA, he only had to pay about $70 of the more than $600 expense to have it removed.

"I went home and called everyone I knew," Tom said. "You can be sure I let my friends know how the ACA saved my life and saved me money. Without insurance, I know I would have waited ... until it was too late."

Obamacare reduces health-care costs for you and America by preventing diseases before they require emergency care. For example, Boston Children's Hospital has a program that sends community health workers into patients' homes to reduce the environmental triggers of asthma. The program has saved $1.46 in health-care costs for every $1 invested. More importantly, 60 percent fewer people were rushed to the emergency room for asthma. The number of asthma sufferers admitted to the hospital fell by 80 percent.[34]

Why You Really *Do* Want Illegal Aliens to Go to Free Health Centers

As mentioned in chapter 2, hospital care is the largest single component of US health-care costs. In 2011, there were 136 million visits emergency room visits, up from 115 million in 2005 and 108 million in 2000. If the number of visits can be lowered, then health care will cost less for everyone. [35]

Nearly 20 percent went for broken bones, sprains, and other musculoskeletal conditions. Another 12 percent went for abdominal pains, headaches, and other general pains. Nearly 8 percent went for cuts, burns, and abcesses. Many of these conditions could be treated as effectively at a lower-cost urgent care or retail clinic.[36]

Why did they go? More than half (54.5 percent) went because their medical problem required hospital treatment. One out of five were told to go by their doctor, and 8.9 percent arrived by ambulance.

However, the other half (46.3 percent) went simply because they really had no other place to go. This lack of access to health care went up to 62 percent for those who weren't insured. A shocking 17.7 percent went because their primary care physician *is* the emergency room.[37]

That's the result of a disturbing trend. Between 1988 and 1996, the number of working people with employer-sponsored insurance plans dropped from 72 percent to 58 percent. During the same time, the number of emergency room visits increased 25 percent. That is more than a coincidence.

The problem has only grown worse. Today, there are twenty-one million immigrants who are not United States citizens. (Only US citizens can apply for Obamacare, although immigrants can apply after five years of legal residency.) Eleven million immigrants are undocumented, commonly known as illegal aliens.

Where do they go for health care? The emergency room of the local hospital. More than 15 percent of emergency room patients were uninsured. The emergency room is the portal of entry for as many as three of every four uninsured patients admitted to the nation's hospitals, according to a 1996 study by the American Hospital Association (AHA).

Hospitals cannot legally turn the uninsured away, thanks to the 1986 federal Emergency Medical Treatment and Labor Act (EMTALA). This law only applies to hospitals that accept Medicare funding, but that's 98 percent of them. It requires hospitals to evaluate and stabilize anyone who shows up at the emergency room, regardless of ability to pay or legal status. If the hospital has a special facility, like a burn unit, they must accept transfers of all patients.

Why did Congress pass EMTALA? The law was passed to keep hospitals from "dumping" uninsured and poor patients onto public hospitals. These patients were two times more likely to die than non-transferred patients, and 24 percent were transferred while still in an unstable condition.

Caring for the uninsured cost hospitals a staggering $10 billion in 1996, according to the AHA study. In the past, hospitals simply shifted the cost to people who had insurance. However, insurance companies got wise and found ways to refuse to pay.[38]

The emergency Medicaid fund reimburses hospitals for some of this treatment. It costs you and other taxpayers $2 billion a year. California alone received half the $2 billion because it has the highest influx of undocumented immigrants. Six other states are also hit especially hard: New York, Texas, Florida, North Carolina, Arizona, and Illinois. [39]

Most of the $2 billion (82 percent) goes toward delivering babies who automatically become US citizens. The rest pays for injuries, kidney failure, and heart conditions.[40]

Obamacare added $11 billion to fund community health centers over five years. These 8,500 centers serve 22 million people. Of those, 40 percent are uninsured, while 38 percent have Medicaid. They are set up to treat everyone, including illegal immigrants, before they require expensive emergency room care. The law also boosted funding for the National Health Service Corps, which helps bring primary care services to underserved populations.

To pay for this, hospitals agreed to a $18 billion cut in federal Medicare payments between 2014 and 2020. They knew that the $11 billion in prevention spending would save them $18 billion in lower emergency room care costs. That's a $7 billion savings for you and other taxpayers.[41]

Prevention Is Cheap, But Not Easy

Hospital administrators have seen the studies that show how preventive care in a few basic areas lowers health costs significantly. They already know that their costs would be lowered significantly if these diseases were prevented altogether. They know that all these preventable diseases can be treated effectively if caught in time.

A study from the National Commission on Prevention Priorities found three simple things that could save two million lives and $4 billion annually: daily aspirin use, tobacco cessation support, and alcohol abuse screening. However, imagine the protests if the government tried to mandate them. People would complain about how their civil rights were being trampled.[42]

Another simple prevention technique is the widespread use of vaccines. Although cancer is one of the top five killers, more people die from diseases that could have been prevented with vaccines than from some forms of cancer (breast, prostate, or colorectal), or from suicide, HIV, or car accidents. In other words, vaccines could prevent nearly 50,000 deaths a year. The flu alone adds $87 billion to health-care costs each year.[43]

How Obamacare Prevents Chronic Diseases

Health-care professionals have known for a long time that in order to lower costs, there must be incentives to help people focus on staying well. That includes programs that encourage active lifestyles, smoking cessation, and vaccinations. These are the most cost-effective ways to lower out-of-control health-care spending.

For example, Trust for America's Health studied community health programs that did just that. Preventive programs, such as nutrition counseling, school exercise programs, and nutrition labeling on restaurant menus, reduced diabetes and high blood pressure by 5 percent within the first two years. States could save between $5 to $10 for every dollar invested in these preventive programs.[44]

Most local politicians who want to get elected respond to their constituencies' concerns, as they should. There are few demonstrations demanding that they install programs to help people eat healthier, exercise more, and stop smoking. In fact, if politicians tried to pass laws that did just that, they'd probably be booted right out of office.

Sometimes the federal government has to step in, and that's what the ACA did. It requires that all insurance, including Medicare and Medicaid, provide preventive care for free. Between 2011 and 2013, more than 100 million Americans received no-cost preventive care of some kind. That means no co-pay and no coinsurance, even if the deductible has not yet been reached, for the following tests, screenings, and procedures:

- Colorectal cancer screening for adults over fifty. That means a colonoscopy, which costs $1,000 or more, is free. However, some insurance companies still charge a fee if a polyp is found and removed. They aren't supposed to, but some say it's no longer preventive but is a treatment. Therefore, check with your insurance company ahead of time to make sure they agree it will be free even if a polyp is found and removed.
- Counseling to prevent or treat alcohol misuse, obesity, sexually transmitted diseases, smoking cessation, and diet for those with chronic diseases. Aspirin use is covered if it's to prevent cardiovascular disease for men and women of certain ages.
- HIV (for those age fifteen to sixty-five and those at high risk) and syphilis tests.
- Blood pressure and cholesterol tests for adults of certain ages or high risk.
- Screening for Type 2 diabetes for adults with high blood pressure, alcohol misuse, tobacco use, depression, obesity, and abdominal aortic aneurysm for men of specified ages who smoked.
- Immunization vaccines, which would otherwise cost you $100 or more, are covered for adults: hepatitis A and B, herpes zoster, human papillomavirus, influenza (flu shot), measles, mumps, rubella, meningococcal, pneumococcal, tetanus, diphtheria, pertussis, and varicella.

Women also get the following tests for free:

- Well-woman visits (for women under sixty-five).
- Screening and counseling for domestic and interpersonal violence.

- Sexually active women receive screening for cervical cancer, chlamydia, gonorrhea, and HIV. Contraception, sterilization procedures, and patient education and counseling are free—although certain religious employers are exempt from providing this benefit.
- Pregnant women receive screening for anemia, hepatitis B, gestational diabetes, Rh incompatibility, syphilis, and urinary tract infections; support and counseling for breastfeeding and to stop smoking; and folic acid supplements.
- Women at risk for breast cancer receive breast cancer genetic test counseling and breast cancer chemoprevention counseling.
- Women over thirty receive the human papillomavirus (HPV) DNA test every three years.
- Women over forty receive a mammogram every one to two years.
- Women over sixty receive osteoporosis screening.

Children receive these additional tests for free:

- Behavioral, medical, and oral health assessments; height, weight, and body mass measurements; blood pressure, dyslipidemia (for those at high risk), and tuberculin testing—to be received at the following ages: one to four years, five to ten years, eleven to fourteen years, and fifteen to seventeen years.
- Newborns: Screenings for hearing disorders, hypothyroidism, PKU, and sickle cell anemia. Gonorrhea preventive medication for the eyes.
- Up to eleven months: Behavioral, medical, and oral health assessments; height, weight, and body mass measurements; blood pressure screening; iron supplements if at risk for anemia.
- One to four years: Developmental and autism screenings.
- Immunizations: Haemophilus influenza type b, rotavirus, and inactivated poliovirus, the same immunizations as adults except for herpes zoster.
- Vision, hemoglobin, lead, and obesity screening.
- Adolescents: depression screening, alcohol and drug use assessments, sexually transmitted disease prevention counseling and HIV tests for those at high risk, cervical dysplasia screening for sexually active females.
- Fluoride chemoprevention supplements for children without fluoride in their water.[45]

The ACA Encourages Companies to Promote Healthy Lifestyles

In 2013, the ACA allowed companies to penalize employees who don't meet specific standards in criteria such as blood pressure, glucose, or cholesterol. For example, Caesar's Entertainment employees get a $50 per month reduction in their health insurance premiums if they agree to undergo tests in these areas. If they meet the goals, or even improve, they're eligible for an additional $500 bonus per year.

Businesses provide these incentives to encourage their workers to take more responsibility for their health. This not only improves their productivity, but also lowers their employers' health insurance costs. The ACA wants to promote healthier workers to lower the cost of Medicare once they retire.

The Rand Corporation reported that more than two-thirds of companies with fifty or more employees and wellness programs use these incentives. However, many of them complain that the ACA regulations are too relaxed. They allow employees that only try to stop smoking, for example, to get the bonuses—even if their efforts aren't successful.[46]

Lower Your Own Health-Care Costs With Just Four Preventive Steps

Obviously, reducing health-care costs lowers your premiums. Even more importantly, it allows you to keep working until you're sixty-five. Nearly half (47 percent) of currently retired people were forced into retirement early, according to the Employee Benefit Research Institute (EBRI). Of those, 55 percent had to quit because of health problems or disabilities. Another 23 percent had to stay home to take care of a family member's health problems. Most retirees don't plan for these health-care costs, which are the second largest expense in their budgets.

Want more shocking statistics? One in four young adults will be disabled before they retire. The most common causes of preventable disability are cancer, strokes, and heart attacks. Finding and treating these illnesses before they cause a disability allows you to keep working so you can put more money toward an active retirement.[47]

You can lower your risk of Alzheimer's disease by reducing heart disease. That means reducing high blood pressure, high blood cholesterol, excess weight, and diabetes.[48]

To keep it simple, the four most important things you can do to prevent disease are:

1. Exercise the equivalent of running one and a half miles a day.
2. Eat fruits, vegetables, nuts, beans, skinless poultry, fish, and lean meat. Think of food as nutrition for your heart, muscles, and brain.
3. Reduce your weight to within the normal BMI range.
4. Refrain from smoking anything.

If you want to lower your personal health-care costs, and avoid these chronic diseases and the top five causes of death, stay focused on two numbers: 120/80 and the number one. The first is your blood pressure; make sure yours is below it. The second is a ratio between the circumference of your waist and that of your hips. Again, make sure yours is always lower than that. In other words, your waist should be smaller than your hips.[49]

Mental Health Care: How Obamacare Helps

Jonathan Stanley was a college junior when he started running through the streets of New York. He had to get away from the CIA agents whom he believed were after him. After three days, he was captured and sent to Manhattan's Bellevue Hospital. His father found him there in a straitjacket.

Fortunately, Jonathan was successfully diagnosed. He had severe bipolar disorder that could be treated with lithium. Today, he is a successful lawyer and advocate for the mentally ill.

Most of the thirteen million Americans with severe mental illnesses are more similar to Jonathan than they are to those the mass media sensationalizes—the homeless, mass murderers, and serial killers. However, left untreated, those with severe mental illnesses may end up that way.[50]

To help treat this problem, the ACA provided an addition $54.6 million to the Department of Health and Human Services to hire mental health professionals. The funds will go to 221 health centers that serve 450,000 people nationwide. That's part of the 1,300 community health centers serving 21.7 million people. In 2013, they already helped 1.2 million substance abusers and mentally ill people.[51]

Mental illness leads to such widely publicized extremes as homelessness, school or other mass shootings, and serial killings because it is not effectively treated. The mentally ill often receive a patchwork of care, bouncing from psychiatrists to counselors and medical doctors. Many do not even get their mental illness correctly diagnosed.

Effective mental health illness prevention and treatment will solve these widely publicized and seemingly intractable problems by addressing the source, not the symptoms. However, this means mental health assessments and treatments need to be affordable and more widely available.

Obamacare addresses this need by making mental health care one of the ten essential benefits. As discussed in chapter 3, it also rewards health-care providers by integrating behavioral health into treatment of physical health.

The Problem with Mental Illness Treatment Today

The nature of mental illnesses makes it difficult for sufferers to keep jobs. Nearly ten million of those with a serious mental illness could not work. More than a third of them went without treatment. As a result, the correlation between poverty and mental illness is high. More than one out of four living in poverty are mentally ill. That means they are least likely to have employer-sponsored health insurance and most likely to be unable to afford treatment. As a result, many end up on Medicaid. They have to shuttle between many different offices, filling out complicated paperwork, and rarely have the skills or means to do so. Many of those who can't afford health care self-medicate with street drugs or alcohol, becoming addicted.

This leads to many physical health problems, such as heart and lung disease, diabetes, and HIV. They wind up in emergency rooms because they receive little or no care until it becomes too late.

As bad as mental hospitals were in the 1960s, they at least kept the mentally ill off of the streets and out of prison. Today, the public mental health system is poorly funded, outdated, and doesn't work well with medical health providers. To make a long and sad story short, most of the chronically and profoundly mentally ill get no treatment and wind up living on the street to face whatever they get.

Homelessness

Integrating mental health into the nation's health-care system will also address one of the main causes of homelessness. More than 610,000 Americans are homeless. Nearly 40 percent have a mental illness or are addicts. Being homeless, in and of itself, worsens their problems. They suffer untreated diabetes and heart disease, injuries from living outdoors, and traumatic experiences.

Specifically, there are three distinct causes of homelessness:

1. More than a third are in families. They've lost a home and/or job and just need some temporary support so they can get on their feet again.
2. Nearly 20 percent are chronically homeless because of mental illness, physical disability, and addiction.
3. Nearly 10 percent are veterans who suffer from Post-Traumatic Stress Disorder (PTSD), addiction, or war-related injuries. Sadly, half of homeless veterans are disabled.[52]

The homeless cost society by their use of emergency rooms, police action, and jails. A homeless person is in the hospital four days longer per visit than normal. Those four days cost taxpayers an extra $2,414 per visit. A study in Hawaii showed that just 1,751 homeless adults were responsible for 564 hospitalizations costing $4 million. They wound up in psychiatric hospitals 100 times more often than the average.

Many of the homeless wind up in jail. A University of Texas study found that this costs taxpayers $14,480 a year just for overnight stays. If they go to prison for more serious crimes, it costs taxpayers $20,000 a year to keep them off the streets.

Homeless shelters are also expensive. Ten percent of those in shelters are families, but they make up 83 percent of total shelter costs. Because they stay longer and have more needs, they can cost anywhere from $3,184 to $20,031 per stay.[53]

Intervention and prevention would treat the many illnesses of the homeless. More than half (52 percent) of the homeless are both mentally ill and substance abusers (alcoholics and drug addicts). As a result, they also have more of the chronic disease killers, such as heart disease, diabetes, and COPD. They're more likely to have contagious diseases like HIV, hepatitis C, and sexually transmitted diseases. Overdose is the number one cause of death.[54]

Veterans who are homeless have a host of other problems, as well. First, they are homeless longer—six years versus four for the average homeless person. There are 62 percent who are chronically homeless (at least two years). That's because they have other serious diseases that contribute to their inability to get off the streets. Nearly three out of four (75 percent) are addicted to drugs or alcohol, 55 percent are mentally ill, and 61 percent have a chronic disease. Sadly, nearly a third (32 percent) have all three health problems.[55]

Mass Shootings and Serial Killers

Mass shootings, such as the one at Sandy Hook Elementary in 2012, receive a lot of media attention, but the true cause is rarely discussed. They are often blamed on everything from today's permissive society to lack of gun control. However, when you track down the actual cases, it's clear it's a result of undiagnosed, untreated, or poorly treated mental illness.

Since 1976, there have been about twenty mass murders a year. J. Reid Meloy, Ph.D, is a forensic psychologist who has studied mass murders over the last fifteen years. He found that mass murderers often have both mental disorders and personality disorders. The mental illnesses range from chronic psychotic disturbances, schizophrenia, and major depression to bipolar disorders and other paranoid disorders. The personality disorders include antisocial, paranoid, narcissistic, and schizoid traits.[56]

Although not judged insane by the courts, mass murderers suffer from poorly treated paranoia and narcissistic personality disorders. That means they are suspicious, self-centered, grandiose, and without empathy for others.

Like mass murderers, serial killers get a lot of media attention but are rarely judged insane by the court because they don't have outright psychosis and schizophrenia. That means they don't kill people because they are obeying orders from voices only they can hear.

However, serial killers suffer from many of the same personality disorders as mass murderers. In addition, they are often psychopaths. That means they seek the sensation of stalking that leads to murder, they have no remorse, and they are control freaks. What makes this personality disorder even more confusing is that psychopaths can be very charming to get what they want. As their need to control increases, this charm leads to manipulation, intimidation, and then violence.

It's clear that if more were done to identify and successfully treat these severely mentally ill people, there would be fewer mass shootings and serial killers. Instead, we are left feeling helpless or arguing over ineffective means of preventing violence, such as gun control. What if there were a way to screen for potential psychopaths before they killed?

Surprisingly, there is an easy-to-use questionnaire that does just that. The Psychopathy Check List Revised (PCL-R) was created by Dr. Robert Hare. He led the modern research effort to develop a series of assessment tools to evaluate the personality traits and behaviors attributable to psychopaths.

Although not all psychopaths are serial killers, and all serial killers are not psychopaths, those that are can be especially dangerous. Violent offenders who are psychopaths have the ability to assault, rape, and murder without the normal human concern for legal, moral, or social consequences. They don't value human life and are extremely callous with their victims. The worst are sexually motivated serial killers, who repeatedly target, stalk, assault, and kill without any remorse.

Thanks to Dr. Hare's tool, these extremely dangerous offenders can be quickly identified by police. Their traits are very predictable, which can help with linking them to crime scene investigations.

Once identified, their narcissism, selfishness, and vanity can be exploited to prosecute them. For example, they will reveal themselves to officers who praise their intelligence, cleverness, and skill in evading capture. This may assist law enforcement in understanding and identifying serial murderers. However, it would be better if these existing screening tools were used before a crime was committed.[57]

Four Solutions Obamacare Provides

The ACA improves treatment for the mentally ill in four ways:

1. It makes mental health treatment more affordable. An astonishing 5.5 million people without health insurance are both mentally ill and poor enough to qualify for Medicaid. That's 17.5 percent of the total thirty-two million uninsured that Obamacare wants to get signed up. Even more will gain access through the health exchanges and receive subsidies.

2. Clinics that focus on the challenge of treating mentally ill substance abusers can reduce emergency room use, according to recent studies. They succeed by integrating medical with behavioral health care. The ACA provides $50 million to create more of these focused integrated care health centers.[58]

3. It mandates that mental health and substance abuse treatment are included in the ten essential benefits. That means all insurance plans must provide this coverage. They can't cut off treatment, no matter how much it costs, because there are no more annual or lifetime limits. They also can no longer deny anyone insurance for preexisting mental conditions, alcoholism, or drug addiction. Sufferers of these diseases don't have to worry that seeking treatment will one day be used against them as a reason for denial of insurance.

4. It creates an integrated care system that is critical for treating both mental illness and addiction. Medicaid can designate a hospital or doctor's office to coordinate care for the patient. It also provides funding for the community-based centers that treat those without access to even Medicaid. It funds training for all medical staff to recognize and treat these complicated and chronic diseases. It also creates the Accountable Care Organizations that can include mental health and addiction counselors, as mentioned in chapter 3.

Warning: Some States May Lose Their Current Mental Health Funding

States that aren't expanding Medicaid may find the federal funding for all mental health and substance abuse treatment being cut back. That's because federal funding for these programs has been consolidated with Medicaid. It's possible that some states will only receive funding for inpatient and outpatient care, and not for screening as part of primary care, community care, and partial hospitalization.

While mental health care is one of the ten essential benefits, states have some leeway in how they define it. Some may only recommend to insurance companies that inpatient treatment is covered. Others will insist that mental health screenings in primary care visits are covered as well.

Furthermore, insurance companies have discretion on how much mental health coverage they offer. For example, they can limit the number of psychotherapy visits per year. Many will only cover services offered by qualified psychiatrists or those with PhDs.

Even if you don't currently need mental health care, it's a good idea to check the fine print in any health plan you choose—just in case. Many mental illnesses, such as bipolar disorder, schizophrenia, and borderline personality disorder, don't manifest until later in life. Many life events, such as job loss, divorce, or death of a loved one, can trigger depression. Receiving a DUI (driving under the influence) can uncover alcoholism that requires treatment. It's better to know what your insurance covers before an upsetting diagnosis of mental illness occurs.[59]

How the ACA's Mental Health Benefits Help You

Do you know someone who is depressed, has a drug or alcohol problem, or who you suspect might have some kind of mental problem? Mental illness is more common than you may think. A 2012 survey found that nearly one out of five adults were diagnosed with a mental illness. Nearly 60 percent never saw a professional or received any treatment for their condition. For almost half of them, they simply couldn't afford it.

The most common mental illness was depression, affecting fifteen million adults. Nearly a third of them went without treatment. As a result, nine million considered suicide, with 1.3 million making an actual attempt.

Nearly one out of four Americans binge drink (five or more drinks at one time in the past month), one out of seven use illegal drugs, and one out of ten smoke pot. All of these figures are higher among those suffering from mental illness.[60]

Imagine if all who went to the doctor for their yearly physical then received screening for alcohol abuse, depression, and smoking. Right then and there, they are sent to detox, receive counseling, or see a pharmacist to get antidepressants or antismoking drugs. When orders from the problem come from a physician, patients might more likely be able to see it as an actual health problem, not "something they should handle on their own." They would get the help they need right away.

Imagine if everyone was screened for these problems at every health visit and referred to someone in their health-care system who would follow up with them. This screening will identify and treat psychotics, those with personality disorders, and others who might have otherwise gone on to commit violent crimes.

The doctor could refer those with severe mental illness to an affiliated specialty mental health clinic located nearby. This specialty clinic would offer treatment for chronic pain, PTSD, and substance abuse. It would also provide exercise classes, nutrition and health education, and even job counseling. It would be staffed with case managers who would integrate all health care for patients with these chronic health issues.

Doctors and counselors would work together, uncovering any emotional blocks the patient has to managing his or her own treatment. Often patients with chronic diseases such as diabetes or those with COPD become frustrated and depressed dealing with such aggravating illnesses. They give up or go into denial. This often triggers medical crises that wind up in the emergency room. The best medical treatment plan in the world won't help if the patient doesn't follow it.

Blending physical and mental health treatment is exactly what the ACA is attempting to do through integrated care, as discussed in chapter 3. In addition, Obamacare covers the costs for these treatments as part of the ten essential benefits.

Medicaid is already helping the homeless by no longer requiring they supply a home address or produce original birth certificates. Agencies that help the homeless receive training, certification, and funding to sign their clients up for Medicaid. The ACA extends Medicaid coverage to young adults who have been in foster care, regardless of where they live or their income.

The ACA helps those regardless of income. Insurance providers cannot refuse coverage or take away your insurance for previous treatment for substance abuse or common mental health diagnoses, such as depression and obsessive-compulsion disorder (OCD). The cost of insurance, and the cost of mental health preventive treatment that it covers, will be cheaper than the cost of treating a mental health crisis with either hospital inpatient treatment ($1,940), psychiatric hospitalization ($905), or detox ($256).[61]

If you are diagnosed with a life-threatening illness, your insurance will cover visits to a mental health professional to help you deal with the emotional reaction to your diagnosis. The same is true with chronic disease diagnoses, like diabetes, heart disease, and COPD.

So many people don't take care of their illnesses because they are in denial. Counseling can help break through this, help them deal with their grief over loss of health, and take proactive steps to manage their illness. This helps avoid expensive crisis care that comes from not managing their illness, such as emergency room treatment for shortness of breath with COPD.

Your insurance must provide coverage for mental health services. People with mental health issues will get treated instead of winding up in jail or homeless—both of which cost society more. As schizophrenics, psychotics, and those with severe personality disorders get screened and treated, there will be fewer incidents of homelessness, mass violence, and serial murders.

Chapter 5: References

1. "The Health Care Law's 10 Essential Benefits," AARP, September 2013. http://www.aarp.org/health/health-insurance/info-08-2013/affordable-care-act-health-benefits.html, accessed September 9, 2014.

2. "Stop Medicare Fraud," US Department of Health and Human Services. http://www.stopmedicarefraud.gov/, accessed September 9, 2014.

3. "Millions with Pre-existing Conditions," Factcheck.com, February 4, 2011. http://www.factcheck.org/2011/02/millions-with-preexisting-conditions/, accessed September 7, 2014. "At Risk: Pre-Existing Conditions Could Affect 1 in 2 Americans," Department of Health and Human Services. http://aspe.hhs.gov/health/reports/2012/pre-existing/index.pdf, accessed September 7, 2014.

4. "Alcohol and Drug Information," National Council on Alcoholism and Drug Dependence, Inc. https://ncadd.org/for-the-media/alcohol-a-drug-information, accessed November 3, 2014.

5. "Cancer Facts and Figures," American Cancer Society. http://www.cancer.org/research/cancerfactsstatistics/cancerfactsfigures2014/index, accessed November 2, 2014.

6. "Alcohol and Drug Information."

7. "Fatty Liver Disease," WebMD. http://www.webmd.com/hepatitis/fatty-liver-disease, accessed November 3, 2014.

8. "About Heart Disease and Stroke," Department of Health and Human Services. http://millionhearts.hhs.gov/abouthds/cost-consequences.html, accessed June 17, 2015.

9. "Epidemiology of the EBD," Centers for Disease Control and Prevention. http://www.cdc.gov/ibd/ibd-epidemiology.htm, accessed November 2, 2014.

10. Amy Norton, "More Americans Getting Pacemakers," Reuters, September 26, 2012. http://www.reuters.com/article/2012/09/26/us-more-americans-getting-pacemakers-idUSBRE88P1LN20120926, accessed November 2, 2014.

11. "Kidney Facts and Figures," Centers for Disease Control and Prevention. http://www.cdc.gov/diabetes/pubs/pdf/kidney_factsheet.pdf, accessed November 2, 2014.

12. "Rheumatoid Arthritis," Centers for Disease Control and Prevention. http://www.cdc.gov/arthritis/basics/rheumatoid.htm, accessed November 2, 2014.

13. "Stroke Facts," Centers for Disease Control and Prevention. http://www.cdc.gov/stroke/facts.htm, accessed November 2, 2014.

14. "Introduction to Intellectual Disabilities," The ARC. http://www.thearc.org/page .aspx?pid=2448, accessed November 3, 2014.

15. "Obesity Facts," Centers for Disease Control and Prevention. http://www.cdc.gov/ obesity/data/adult.html, accessed November 2, 2014; Cynthia L. Ogden, PhD; Margaret D. Carroll, MSPH; Brian K. Kit, MD, MPH; Katherine M. Flegal, PhD, "Prevalence of Childhood and Adult Obesity in the United States, 2011–2012," *Journal of the American Medical Association*, February 26, 2014. http://jama.jamanetwork. com/article.aspx?articleid=1832542, accessed November 3, 2014.

16. Stephanie J. Verntura, M.A., Sally C. Curtin, M.A., Joyce C. Abma, Ph.D., Division of Vital Statistics, and Stanley K. Henshaw, Ph.D., The Guttmacher Institute, "Estimated Pregnancy Rates and Rates of Pregnancy Outcomes of the United States, 1990–2008," *National Vital Statistics Report*, Volume 60, Number 7, June 20, 2012. http://www.cdc.gov/nchs/data/nvsr/nvsr60/nvsr60_07.pdf, accessed November 3, 2014. "Michigan's High Risk Pool Program Presumptive Eligibility List of Pre-Existing Conditions," http://www.michigan.gov/documents/dleg/Pre-Ex_330602_7. pdf, accessed November 3, 2014. "Pre-Existing Condition Exclusions," Blue Cross and Blue Shield of Illinois. http://www.ilhealthagents.com/bluecross-blueshield-illinois/pre-existing-conditions.html, accessed November 3, 2014.

17. Phil Galewitz, "Millions Previously Denied Insurance Coverage Because of Health Problems Look to Online Marketplaces," Kaiser Health News, September 30, 2013. http://kaiserhealthnews.org/news/preexisting-condition-consumers-insurance-obamacare-marketplaces/, accessed November 4, 2014.

18. Jeffrey Brenner, MD, "Addressing the One Percent: An Interview with Jeffrey Brenner, MD," *Camden Coalition*, November 6, 2012. http://www.camdenhealth.org/ addressing-the-one-percent-an-interview-with-jeffrey-brenner-md/, November 5, 2014.

19. Sophie Novack, "Is Obamacare Living Up to Its Pre-existing Promise?" *National Journal*, June 23, 2014. http://www.nationaljournal.com/health-care/is-obamacare-living-up-to-its-preexisting-conditions-promise-20140623, accessed November 3, 2014.

20. Igor Volsky, "No, Obamacare Won't Cover Every Drug—Just Like Every Other Insurance Policy," ThinkProgress.org, December 10, 2013. http://thinkprogress.org/ health/2013/12/10/3042741/drugs-obamacare-coverage/, accessed November 3, 2014.

21. "The 10 Most Expensive Medical Procedures," *Healthcare Business & Technology*, April 16, 2012. http://www.healthcarebusinesstech.com/the-10-most-expensive-medical-procedures/

22. "Under the Affordable Care Act, 105 Million No Longer Face Lifetime Health Benefits," ASPE.hhs.gov, March 2012. http://aspe.hhs.gov/health/reports/2012/LifetimeLimits/ib.shtml, accessed October 31, 2014.

23. Michelle Andrews, "Caps on Coverage; A Big Point of Conflict," *New York Times*, January 27, 2010.

24. "National Prematurity Awareness Month," Centers for Disease Control and Prevention. http://www.cdc.gov/features/prematurebirth/, accessed November 1, 2014. "Preterm Birth," CDC. http://www.cdc.gov/reproductivehealth/maternalinfanthealth/PretermBirth.htm, accessed June 17, 2015.

25. Scott D. Smith, "Million-Dollar Miracles," *Minnesota Medicine*, April 2006. http://www.minnesotamedicine.com/Past-Issues/Past-Issues-2006/April-2006/Feature-April-2006, accessed November 1, 2014.

26. Michelle Andrews, "Rate of Premature Births Fall as Health Law Provisions Begin to Take Effect," Kaiser Health News, November 7, 2014. http://kaiserhealthnews.org/news/rate-of-premature-births-fall-as-health-law-provisions-begin-to-take-effect/, accessed November 1, 2014.

27. "Cancer in Children and Adults," National Cancer Institute, http://www.cancer.gov/cancertopics/factsheet/Sites-Types/childhood, accessed October 31, 2014.

28. David Linney, "Managing Your Health Insurance Lifetime Limits," *Hemaware*. http://www.hemaware.org/story/managing-your-health-insurance-lifetime-limits, accessed October 31, 2014. "Hemophilia Causes," *Mayo Clinic*. http://www.mayoclinic.org/diseases-conditions/hemophilia/basics/causes/con-20029824, accessed June 17, 2015. "HIV/AIDS," National Hemophilia Foundation, https://www.hemophilia.org/Bleeding-Disorders/Blood-Safety/HIV/AIDS, accessed June 17, 2015. Bruce Goldfarb and Sarah Aldrige, "Hepatitis C and Hemophilia," *Hemaware*, May 23 2011. http://www.hemaware.org/story/hepatitis-c-and-hemophilia, accessed June 17, 2015.

29. "Sepsis Data Report," Centers for Disease Control and Prevention. http://www.cdc.gov/sepsis/datareports/index.html, accessed November 2, 2014.

30. Joanne Volk, "Affordable Care Act's Ban on Lifetime Limits Has Ended Martin Addie's Coverage Circus," Georgetown University Health Policy Institute, November

14, 2012. http://ccf.georgetown.edu/all/affordable-care-acts-ban-on-lifetime-limits-has-ended-martin-addies-coverage-circus/, accessed November 21, 2014.

31. Mark Landler and Michael D. Shear, "Obama Says Young Adults Push Health Care Enrollment Above Targets," *New York Times*, April 18, 2014. http://www.nytimes.com/2014/04/18/us/obama-says-young-adults-push-health-care-enrollment-above-targets.html, accessed November 21, 2014.

32. "The Impact of Lifetime Limits," PricewaterhouseCoopers, March 2009. http://www.amcp.org/WorkArea/DownloadAsset.aspx?id=12211, accessed June 17, 2015.

33. "Lifetime and Annual Limits," Health and Human Services. http://www.hhs.gov/healthcare/rights/limits/, accessed November 21, 2014. "Annual Limits," CMS.gov. http://www.cms.gov/CCIIO/Programs-and-Initiatives/Health-Insurance-Market-Reforms/Annual-Limits.html, accessed June 17, 2015.

34. Sharon Begley, "Think Preventive Medicine Will Save Money? Think Again," Reuters, January 29, 2013. http://www.reuters.com/article/2013/01/29/us-preventive-economics-idUSBRE90S05M20130129, accessed November 4, 2014.

35. "Emergency Department Visits," Centers for Disease Control and Prevention http://www.cdc.gov/nchs/fastats/emergency-department.htm, accessed June 17, 2015.

36. Robin M. Weinick, Rachel M. Burns, and Ateev Mehrotra, "How Many Emergency Department Visits Could be Managed at Urgent Care and Retail Clinics?" *Health Affairs*. 2010 September; 29(9): 1630–1636. http://content.healthaffairs.org/content/29/9/1630.long, accessed June 17, 2015.

37. Renee M. Gindi, PhD, Robin A. Cohen, PhD, and Whitney K. Kirzinger, MPH, "Emergency Room Use Among Adults Aged 18–64: Early Release of Estimates From the National Health Interview Survey, January-June 2011," Centers for Disease Control and Prevention, May 2012. http://www.cdc.gov/nchs/data/nhis/earlyrelease/emergency_room_use_january-june_2011.pdf, accessed November 4, 2014.

38. Joseph Zibulewsky, MD, "The Emergency Medical Treatment and Active Labor Act (EMTALA): What It Is and What It Means for Physicians," National Institute of Health, October 2001. http://www.ncbi.nlm.nih.gov/pmc/articles/PMC1305897/, accessed November 4, 2014.

39. Phil Galewitz and Kaiser Health News, "How Undocumented Immigrants Sometimes Receive Medicaid Treatment," *PBS NewsHour*, February 13, 2013. http://www

.pbs.org/newshour/rundown/how-undocumented-immigrants-sometimes-receive-medicaid-treatment/, accessed November 4, 2014.

40. C. Annette DuBard, MD, MPH, Mark W. Massing, MD, MPH, PhD, "Trends in Emergency Medicaid Expenditures for Recent and Undocumented Immigrants," *Journal of the American Medical Association*, March 14, 2007, Volume 297, No. 10. http://jama.jamanetwork.com/article.aspx?articleid=206014, accessed November 4, 2014.

41. Julie Appleby, "FAQ: Obamacare and Coverage for Immigrants," Kaiser Health News, September 19, 2013. http://kaiserhealthnews.org/news/health-care-immigrants/, accessed November 4, 2014.

42. "Prevention Saves Lives as Well as Money, New Research Confirms," Medscape, 2010. http://www.medscape.com/viewarticle/735245, accessed July 29, 2014.

43. "The Impact of Chronic Diseases on Healthcare Prevention," For a Healthier America. http://www.forahealthieramerica.com/ts/prevention-adult-immunization.html, accessed July 29, 2014.

44. Joshua T. Cohen, PhD, Peter J. Neumann, ScD, and Milton C. Weinstein, PhD, "Does Preventive Care Save Money?" *New England Journal of Medicine*, February 14, 2008. http://www.nejm.org/doi/full/10.1056/NEJMp0708558, accessed July 29, 2014. Megan Greenhall, "Disease Prevention Called a Better Bet," *The Washington Post*, July 18, 2008. http://www.washingtonpost.com/wp-dyn/content/article/2008/07/17/AR2008071700990.html, accessed June 17, 2015.

45. "What Are My Preventive Care Benefits?" Healthcare.gov. https://www.healthcare.gov/preventive-care-benefits, accessed July 29, 2014.

46. Stephanie Armour, "CEOs Say Federal Limits Are Ailing Wellness Programs," *Wall Street Journal*, September 4, 2014.

47. Nevin Adams, "Work 'Forces'," EBRI, May 2, 2014. https://ebriorg.wordpress.com/category/retirement/early-retirees/, accessed November 4, 2014.

48. "Prevention," Mayo Clinic. http://www.mayoclinic.org/diseases-conditions/alzheimers-disease/basics/prevention/con-20023871, accessed November 4, 2014.

49. Interview with Dr. Jay McFarland, DC, Advanced Bank Pain and Injury Center, Phoenix Arizona, December 5, 2014.

50. Eric S. Lander and Louis V. Gerstner Jr., "Private Money Pays Off for Medicine," *Wall Street Journal*, August 11, 2014.

51. "HHS Awards $54.6 Million in Affordable Care Act Mental Health Services Funding," US Department of Health & Human Services, July 2014. http://www.hhs.gov/news/press/2014pres/07/20140731a.html, accessed July 31, 2014.

52. "The State of Homelessness in America 2014," National Alliance to End Homelessness. http://b.3cdn.net/naeh/d1b106237807ab260f_qam6ydz02.pdf, accessed July 31, 2014.

53. Brooke Spellman, Jill Khadduri, Brian Sokol, Josh Leopold, Abt Associates, "Costs Associated With First-Time Homelessness for Families and Individuals," US Department of Housing and Urban Development, March 2010. http://www.huduser.org/portal//publications/pdf/Costs_Homeless.pdf, accessed December 6, 2014.

54. "Integrated Quick Care Guide," National Healthcare for the Homeless Council, September 2013. http://www.nhchc.org/wp-content/uploads/2013/10/integrated-care-quick-guide-sept-2013.pdf, accessed July 31, 2014.

55. "National Survey of Homeless Veterans in 100,000 Homes Campaign Communities," Veterans Administration, November 2011. http://www.va.gov/HOMELESS/docs/NationalSurveyofHomelessVeterans_FINAL.pdf, accessed December 6, 2014.

56. J. Reid Meloy, Ph.D., "Seven Myths of Mass Murder," *Psychology Today*, April 21. 2014. https://www.psychologytoday.com/blog/the-forensic-files/201404/seven-myths-mass-murder, accessed June 17, 2015.

57. Robert J. Morton, "Serial Murders: Multi-Disciplinary Perspectives for Investigators," FBI, August 29, 2005. http://www.fbi.gov/stats-services/publications/serial-murder, accessed July 31, 2014

58. "Integrated Care Quick Guide: Integrating Behavioral Health and Primary Care in the HCH Setting," National Healthcare for the Homeless Council, September 2013. http://www.nhchc.org/wp-content/uploads/2013/10/integrated-care-quick-guide-sept-2013.pdf, accessed November 5, 2014. Bevin Croft and Susan L. Parish, "Care Integration in the Patient Protection and Affordable Care Act: Implications for Behavioral Health," ACGOV.org, February 28, 2012. https://www.acgov.org/board/district3/documents/2012-07-23ACA-ImplicationsBehavioralHealth.pdf, accessed December 6, 2014.

59. John M. Grohol, PsyD, "An Update on How the U.S. Affordable Care Act Impacts Mental Health Care," PsychCentral, November 1, 2013. http://psychcentral

.com/blog/archives/2013/11/01/an-update-on-how-the-u-s-affordable-care-act-impacts-mental-health-care/, accessed July 31, 2014.

60. "Results from the 2013 National Survey on Drug Use and Health: Mental Health Findings," US Department of Health and Human Services, September 2014. http://www.samhsa.gov/data/sites/default/files/NSDUHmhfr2013/NSDUHmhfr2013.pdf, accessed December 6, 2014.

61. "Linking Housing and Health Care Works for Chronically Homeless Persons," US Department of Housing and Urban Development, Summer 2012. http://www.huduser.org/portal/periodicals/em/summer12/highlight3.html, accessed July 31, 2014.

Chapter 6

BUY THE BEST HEALTH INSURANCE FOR YOU

Buying health insurance is primarily a financial decision. Before you choose a plan, you've got to weigh how likely you are to get sick versus your projected income. This means you've got to be an odds-maker on your own health.

Most people just want the cheapest health insurance they can find. They often only look at the premium and go for the one with the lowest monthly payment. This decision will probably cost you more if you need medical care. That's because there are many hidden fees in health insurance. Your total payment is not just the premium, but also includes the deductible, coinsurance, and co-payment. You need to choose the level for each type of payment.

Unfortunately, all these choices make picking health-care insurance very complicated. Options with examples are indicated below. They start from the least expensive (and least protection) to the most expensive (and most protection).

Review these choices, but before you take action, check to see if you qualify for a subsidy. (Find out how in chapter 7.) More than half of the people who *could* have gotten subsidies on the ACA exchanges didn't even apply. That would apply to you if, for example, if you were single and made less than $46,680 in 2015.

Apply for an Exemption

Don Nickerson is 62 and filed for bankruptcy last year because of credit card debt. He lost his home and his job and now can only find part-time work. He's not obligated to get health insurance because he doesn't have enough income to file taxes. However, he does qualify for Medicaid in his state. He should apply on the marketplace to get free preventive care.

Even if you are exempt from the penalty, you might still want to get insurance in order to protect yourself from the financial risks of being without insurance.

Check if any of the following exemptions apply to you:

- Don't make enough to pay income taxes.
- Your premiums would be more than 8.05 percent of your income.
- Uninsured for less than three months.
- In jail.
- Don't live in the United States.
- A member of a Native American tribe, a health-care sharing ministry, or a religious sect that objects to any form of insurance.

Since 2010, HHS has added the following exemptions for those experiencing special hardship conditions. You can file for a hardship exemption if you were:

- Unable to find insurance with a premium of less than 8 percent of your income.
- Homeless.
- Evicted or faced eviction or foreclosure in the past six months.
- The recipient of a shut-off notice from a utility company.
- A close family member of someone who recently passed away.
- A victim of domestic violence that prevented you from getting health insurance.
- Earning 138 percent or below the poverty level and your state didn't expand Medicaid.
- Bankrupt (filed in the last six months).
- A victim of fire or flood damage to your residence.
- In debt due to medical expenses or from caring for a sick family member.
- Denied Medicaid or CHIP for your child, and someone else was supposed to pay for medical support but didn't.
- Eligible for subsidies, but the insurance company didn't give them to you and so you were without insurance.
- Waiting for the results of an appeal that decided you were eligible for a plan on the exchange.
- Taken off of your previous insurance plan by the insurance company.
- Unable to obtain insurance for some other reason that was approved by HHS.

If you qualify for a hardship exemption, you can apply for low-cost catastrophic insurance. It covers hospitalization and preventive care but has a high deductible. The list of exemptions changes from time to time, so go to Healthcare.gov/exemptions before filing.

Penalty vs. No Penalty

Alex Lawson is a self-employed contractor. He makes $45,000 a year, but most of it goes to child support from a previous marriage. He wasn't worried about paying the ACA penalty and so never got around to getting health insurance.

Two weeks ago, Alex broke his arm when he fell playing basketball. He thought it was sprained. That night, it began to hurt so bad that he drove himself to the emergency room. His arm was broken, and the doctors had to put it in a cast.

When Alex received the hospital bill, he was shocked to find out the charge was $2,500. He learned he'll also have to pay for follow-up doctor visits and physical therapy to regain full use of his hand, which he must have to go back to work. Now he's scrambling to find the money and keep up with his child support payments.

The tax penalty is not affordable for most. In 2016, the tax is 2.5 percent of your Adjusted Gross Income (AGI). The first $10,150 of your income is subject to the tax. However, no matter your income, you'll still pay a minimum, and you won't pay more than the maximum. The minimum is $695 for each uninsured adult plus $347.50 for each uninsured child. However, if you have a lot of uninsured people in your family, your minimum payment won't be more than $2,085 per household.

The maximum is the national average premium cost of purchasing the "Bronze" health insurance plan on the exchange. If your tax is that high, you may as well buy the insurance.

If this makes no sense, here's another way to look at it:

- The tax is 2.5 percent of your AGI above $10,150, but no lower than the minimum and no higher than the maximum.
- The minimum = $695 per adult + $347.50 per child up to $2,085 per household.
- The maximum = the cost of the Bronze plan.

The tax rate rises with the rate of inflation, as measured by the Consumer Price Index (CPI).[1]

Buy Catastrophic Insurance

If you are under thirty or can't find insurance for less than 8.05 percent of your income, you can buy a special high-deductible *catastrophic* plan. It only covers three primary care visits and the preventive services required by the ACA. The deductible is equal to the out-of-pocket maximum, which was $6,600 for individuals and $13,200 for a family in 2015. After that, the insurance company pays 100 percent. As the name says, it will protect your life savings from a truly catastrophic medical bill.

Buy Short-Term Insurance

You can get short-term insurance any time, even outside of the enrollment period. These plans are for time periods of twelve months or less. They are designed to provide coverage until you can sign up for insurance at the next enrollment period. They don't have to comply with the ACA, so offer limited benefits, and don't usually cover preexisting conditions. These plans don't offer subsidies, but are usually less expensive than regular health insurance. However, you still have to pay the ACA tax penalty if you were insured for less than nine months out of any year.

A good place to find short-term insurance, as well as vision, dental, and other health insurance, is GetInsured.com or EHealthInsurance.com. These websites guide you through the steps to shop and compare plans. They give you an estimated quote based on your age and other personal information. Once you decide on a plan, they'll connect you with the provider. They also have phone numbers to call if you're more comfortable with that: GetInsured.com is (866) 602-8466 and EHealthInsurance is (844) 229-4337.

Get Insurance from Your Employer

This is usually the best option if your company offers it because most employers subsidize the cost. Most companies only offer one plan, but you can choose between single or family coverage. Many also offer coverage for same-sex and/or opposite sex domestic partners. Nearly 150 million non-elderly people have plans through their employer.

Roughly two-thirds of the employer plans comply with the ACA. The ones that don't are grandfathered in, which means the employees have had them since 2010.

Only 55 percent of companies still offer health benefits, down from 61 percent in 2012. Most that don't offer benefits are small companies (three to nine employees), while all the companies with one thousand or more workers do offer them. If you absolutely must have company-sponsored insurance, look for a job with companies with more than one thousand employees.

You may have to wait until you're eligible. Most companies make you work for a certain period of time, although the ACA limits the waiting period to no more than ninety days. You must also work a minimum number of hours to be eligible.

A third of the companies also requires you to take a risk assessment that asks questions about your medical history, current health, and lifestyle. This personal information tells them who the high-risk employees are. Many will pay you as much as $500 to take the test. You might have to pay higher insurance costs if you're a smoker or have other high-risk attributes.

More than half of the large companies will offer biometric screening. It measures risk factors such as weight, cholesterol, and blood pressure. A few require you to take the exam in order to be eligible for insurance. Nearly 10 percent will reward or penalize you based on the results.

To help you become healthier (and cost the insurance company less), most companies offer a wellness program. This ranges from a wellness newsletter to personal health coaching. Many will offer a financial incentive, such as a gift card, to participate.

The employee share of the insurance cost is rising. In fact, workers' premiums have more than doubled, as mentioned in chapter 4. Therefore, it still might make sense to compare your employer's plan with plans on the exchange to see if it costs you less with the subsidy. This is more likely the case if you work for a small company.

Types of Employer Plans

Your employer will offer you one of the four following types of plans:

PPO (Preferred Provider Organization). Half of all employees are covered by PPOs. You must use a provider in the network or pay a higher cost.

HMO (Health Maintenance Organization). You are assigned a primary care doctor within the organization. He or she must refer you to any specialist. You won't be covered at all if you don't follow this procedure. This is usually the lowest-cost option, but only 13 percent of employees are covered by HMOs. Many people dislike the restrictions.

HSA (Health Savings Account) Eligible. These are high-deductible PPOs that allow you to set some income aside, tax-free, to pay for medical expenses. They usually have low premiums. Roughly one out of five employees have chosen this option.

Indemnity. You can choose any doctor you want, but you usually have to submit the claims yourself. These are usually the most expensive plans since they provide the most freedom of choice. Only 1 percent of employees are covered by this type of plan.[2]

You can find out about the plans offered from your human resources benefits administrator.

Buy Private Insurance on Your Own

Buying your own health insurance can seem daunting because it's very complicated. Sometimes it seems downright overwhelming, but that's only because you're not yet familiar with the terminology and how it applies to you. The overall goal is to get the best coverage for your individual health needs for the lowest cost.

Fortunately, in chapter 4 you were introduced to what insurance is and how it works. You already know the difference between premiums, deductibles, coinsurance, and copayments. Below is more information you need to make the best choices.

Which Type of Plan Is Best for You?

Just like employer insurance, private insurance offers the same types of plans. This is the most important decision if you already have relationships with certain doctors. You'll want to get honest about what your possible health needs will be before comparing the types of plans. Here are the pros and cons of each:

PPO (Preferred Provider Organization). PPOs offer fewer choices of healthcare providers than an indemnity plan does, but more than a HMO. Most doctors are aligning with just one PPO and hospital network. Your favorite doctors may not be with the same PPOs, and then you've got a decision to make. If you have specific chronic illnesses, you'll want to go with the PPO that the best specialist is affiliated with, and it may not be the same PPO that your primary care doctor is with. If you have small children or elderly family members on your plan, you might want the PPO with the closest emergency room. If you have chronically ill children, you'll want to go with the PPO that has a children's hospital in its network.

HMO (Health Maintenance Organization). HMOs offer the least choice. If you're relatively healthy, this will be the least expensive option for you. If you don't live near the HMO, it will be very inconvenient.

Indemnity. If you absolutely must have two doctors that are in different PPOs, then this is the best way to go. Otherwise, you'll save money in another plan.

HSA (Health Savings Account) Eligible. Since these are high-deductible plans, they are good only if you have enough income to pay your medical costs until you hit the deductible. If that's the case, it's a great way to lower your tax bill by investing pretax dollars. Just as importantly, all the earnings from the investment are tax-free.

Three Ways to Buy Private Insurance

Most people start with a health insurance agent or broker because he or she personally guides them through the steps. What's the difference between an agent and a broker? The agent works for a specific insurance company, while a broker can introduce you to any company. If you already know the insurance company you want, then the agent can probably get you a better price and can more easily facilitate any plan changes. If you really aren't sure, then a broker can help you shop plans for the best fit. You might end up paying more with a broker than with an agent for that specific plan, but you might also find a better plan for less by shopping around. Both agents and brokers receive commissions from the insurance company, so that may increase the price of either plan above what you'd pay if you did all the sleuthing yourself.[3]

How do you find a good agent or broker? Obviously, ask family and friends, but if most of them have insurance from their employers, they won't be any help. In that case, find one through the National Association of Health Underwriters (NAHU). The agents and brokers are licensed and promise to abide by the association's ethics, which require them to keep the customer's best interests in mind when making recommendations. Many have completed college-level courses to become certified and attend NAHU conferences and seminars to stay on top of the latest changes. Each state also requires that they take continuing education classes to retain their license. Find a NAHU agent in your area at http://www.nahu.org/consumer/findagent2.cfm.

You can use GetInsured.com or EHealthInsurance.com to search for the same kind of plans that are on the exchanges. They will also offer the same subsidies.

You can contact the health insurance company directly. If you know your doctor only works with one plan, then this will save you time. Otherwise, researching insurance can be time-consuming because you have to go to each company's website to compare plans.

If you already have private insurance and want to keep your plan, it might not be on the exchange. There were 120 companies in 2014 that did have plans on the exchange. So far, many areas still only have one provider. However, they must still offer you the same subsidies. If you know you want to keep your provider, you may as well go to its website and see which one is the best plan for you.

More and more people are using healthcare.gov to get insurance through the health-care exchanges. It was difficult to use in the beginning, but it's much improved now.

How the Insurance Exchange Works

You can only buy insurance on the exchanges during the open enrollment time. For coverage in 2016, open enrollment is from November 1, 2015 to January 31, 2016. The exact dates change from year-to-year but are typically around that same timeframe.

However, you can visit the exchanges any time to research plans, see if you qualify for a subsidy, and compare doctors, hospitals, and other health providers. You can also use them to see if you qualify for expanded Medicaid, which you can get any time of the year.

The exchanges are run by either your state or HHS, depending on whether your state legislature decided to run its own site. Seventeen states and the District of Columbia manage their own exchanges, while seven states partner with the federal government. If you heard there is a long wait time on the federal exchanges, be assured that it's no longer true.

The exchange guides you through a series of questions to help you find the best plan for you. It defines insurance terms so you know what they are talking about. They do ask some surprisingly personal questions at the beginning, but that's just to get verified. It's really not much different than when you fill out information for a loan.

The federally run exchanges use this four-step process:

1. Create an account. It will ask for your Social Security number, employer's name and address, and your income. Most of us are uncomfortable putting all this personal info into a website. Others don't want the government to get this personal information. However, if you have a Social Security number, the Internal Revenue Service has it anyway.
2. Provide Social Security and income information to see if you qualify for tax credits.
3. Review plans in the four categories (Bronze, Silver, Gold, and Platinum). Each category has different monthly premiums, deductibles, and co-pays. (More on that below.)
4. Enroll in the plan.

Types of Exchange Plans

All plans on the exchanges offer the same level of service. This means they must provide some coverage in each of the ten essential benefits and comply with all other ACA requirements. The out-of-pocket maximum can be no more than $6,600 for an individual plan or $13,200 for a family plan in 2015.

Therefore, your choice will depend on whether the plan includes your preferred doctors and hospitals. Typically, an insurance company will contract with a hospital system and its affiliated doctors and medical practices. Therefore, your first step is to find out which insurance company or companies your doctor is covered by.

After that, your choice will depend on how much you're willing to pay in return for levels of insurance coverage. Each plan offers a different mixture of deductibles, premiums, co-payments, and coinsurance. There are four levels:

Bronze Plan. This insurance pays 60 percent of your medical bills while you pay 40 percent (not including premiums). Bronze plans usually have the lowest premiums since they offer the lowest percentage of coverage. However, they have higher deductibles and coinsurance rates. They are also more likely to be HMOs, which limits the choice of doctors. They are good plans if you are young, healthy, or otherwise know you won't have many medical expenses. However, even if you're healthy, you could still break a leg or have an accident, so make sure you can afford your out-of-pocket expenses without going bankrupt or losing your home.

Silver Plan. This plan pays 70 percent of your health-care costs. You pay 30 percent overall through deductibles, co-payments, and coinsurance. Deductibles tend to be in the $2,000 for singles/$4,000 for families range, and premiums are higher.

Gold Plan. This plan pays 80 percent of your medical costs, while you pay 20 percent through your choice of deductibles, co-pays, and coinsurance rates. Most Gold plans have lower deductibles, but the premiums are higher than for the Bronze plans. There are more PPOs along with HMOs.

Platinum Plan. The insurance company will pick up 90 percent of health-care costs. You pay 10 percent through co-pays, deductibles, and coinsurance. These plans have the lowest deductibles and out-of-pocket maximums. These are good plans if you know your annual medical costs will be higher than your total premiums for the year.

Each level pays a different percentage of medical costs. Keep in mind, however, they all provide the same ten essential benefits, allow you to get the same subsidies, and comply with all ACA regulations. That means they all must provide free preventive care and must pay 100 percent of all medical costs once you've paid the out-of-pocket maximum. The difference in coverage will show up in the premiums, deductibles, and co-pays.

The next section will help you figure out how to choose between these levels of coverage.

Find Your Best Plan Now

Betty Hafler was a sixty-two-year-old receptionist making $44,000 a year. Fortunately, she had been frugal during her life and had saved up $250,000 for retirement. Between this and Social Security, she had enough to retire if she protected her nest egg.

She wanted to keep her primary care physician, so she went with the PPO that covered him. She also knew she would have some medical expenses, so she got a Health Savings Account to reduce her tax bill.

Because of her age and income, she received $100 a month in subsidies. That's because her adjusted gross income after expenses was low, and the cost of a Silver plan (upon which the subsidy is based) was high. She went with a low-deductible Silver plan that had a high out-of-pocket maximum and a reasonable premium. Unless something happened, she wouldn't reach the out-of-pocket but could afford it if necessary. On the other hand, she knew she'd spend more than the deductible in the upcoming year.

The way to evaluate health insurance is to decide how much you can afford in premiums plus the out-of-pocket maximum versus how likely you are to get sick. In general, if you already have a chronic illness, choose a plan with a higher premium but a lower coinsurance and deductible level. If you're very healthy, you can probably risk a low-premium, higher-deductible plan, since you probably won't go to the doctor very much. Ask yourself the following questions.

How Much Medical Expense Can You Comfortably Afford?

Below are the different costs and how to evaluate them:

Co-payment. Evaluate co-payments as you would premiums. If you don't visit the doctor a lot, you can afford a lower premium combined with a higher co-payment.If, on the other hand, you have a chronic illness that requires many doctor visits and medicines, add up those costs. Select a plan where the total co-payment amount saved is more than the higher premium payments. Keep in mind that, under the ACA, co-payments are waived for preventive care like annual wellness exams and mammograms. See chapter 5 for more.

Deductible. Here again, if you're healthy, choose a plan with a low premium and a high deductible. If you've got a chronic illness, you'd probably be better off paying the higher premium to get the lower deductible.

Coinsurance. Once the deductible has been met, the insurance will only pay a certain percentage, called coinsurance. You pay the other percent of the coinsurance. This can get to be pretty expensive if you're in the hospital a lot, so you'll want a high premium, low-deductible plan where the insurance picks up a higher percentage of the coinsurance.

Out-of-pocket maximum. The ACA makes sure you don't wipe out your life savings with coinsurance fees. That's why it limits your total expenses in 2015 to $6,600 individual/$13,200 family. Once you've paid that amount in deductibles, co-payments, coinsurance, and other eligible medical bills, the insurance company picks up 100 percent of the rest.

If you either earn enough or have enough in savings to easily pay the costs, then you will probably want a high-deductible plan. You'll probably pay for all medical costs, but your premium will be lower. Since you have a high deductible, it doesn't really matter what the coinsurance percentage is.

If you are young, and have around $6,500 in savings to protect, you may want to go for the low-deductible plan. Even though your monthly premium will eat up more of your income, you can rest assured that your savings won't be gone in a flash.

If paying the out-of-pocket maximum would mean you lose your house or must declare bankruptcy, then you'll want the lowest-deductible plan with the lowest coinsurance that you can afford. That's because you'll have to pay larger premiums, but it will be worth the peace of mind knowing you won't go homeless if you get in a car accident.

For example, if you are living paycheck to paycheck, a $2,500 hospital visit for a broken arm could force you to miss a few house payments and possibly lose your home. In that case, it might be worth paying a higher premium in return for the lowest deductible and coinsurance.

How Much Did You Spend Last Year on Health Care?

Once you add up how much you spent last year, use it to estimate how much you'll probably spend this year. If it's a lot, you may want a lower-deductible plan so you pay less out of pocket. If you *know* you are planning on having a baby, will need major surgery, or have a chronic illness, then a higher premium will be worth the lower deductible that you know you'll have to pay.

If you know you'll have a lot of doctor visits but may not need hospitalization, then a plan with a low co-payment will save you money. On the other hand, if you need just a single, outpatient surgery that won't require a lot of medication or doctor visits, then you won't care as much about the co-payment, but will definitely want low coinsurance.

Let's say you are very healthy, you're single, and you have $10,000 saved in case of emergencies. You look at plans where you live, and a Bronze plan on the exchange costs $325 a month in premiums. The deductible is $5,000. The coinsurance is 60/40, which means the insurance company pays 60 percent of costs, and the co-pay is $20 per visit and $500 per emergency room visit. However, none of these kick in until after you make the deductible. The out-of-pocket maximum is $6,600. Don't forget, your preventive care is 100 percent covered all the time.

You'll pay $3,900 a year if you never even visit a doctor. If you do get sick, you'll pay $5,000 before any insurance kicks in at all. Once the deductible is paid, you'll pay another $1,600 in coinsurance and co-pays until the out-of-pocket is hit, and the insurance picks up everything. Therefore, your total for the year if you get sick is $10,500, or the total premium of $3,900 plus the $6,600 of out-of-pocket maximum.

On the other hand, suppose you have a chronic illness, you're still single, and still have $10,000 in savings. You know you'll be in and out of the hospital this year. You'd probably want a Platinum plan, which pays 90 percent in coinsurance. It also has a $500 deductible and an out-of-pocket maximum of $1,500. Sounds like a much better deal, right?

It's better, but not by much. The premium is $698 a month, for which you pay $8,376 a year. Add on the $1,500 out-of-pocket, and you'll wind up paying $9,876 in total. This is just $624 less than the Bronze plan. However, if you know you'll be sick, it's worth it.

How Attached Are You to Your Doctor?

If you need to keep your doctor, hospital network, and/or your prescription medicines, then make sure you get a PPO that has him/her in the network. If it doesn't matter, then an HMO will be cheaper.

Are there specific brand-name medications you want to keep? Co-pays and deductibles might be different for your specific drug, or the insurance plan may recommend a generic instead. If you need coverage for a brand name drug, check each health plan's formulary. That's the list of drugs approved by the health insurance company and how much of the price it covers. It can change at any time, depending on negotiations between the insurer, the employer, and drug companies. Formularies typically include both name-brand drugs, which are covered by a patent, and generics, which are cheaper knock-offs that spring up when the patent wears off. You can find the formulary on each health plan's website.

Once you've narrowed it down to two or three plans within a level, you may want to compare them based on the following specifics: How many days does the plan cover in the hospital? How many visits to a physical therapist, mental health professional, or chiropractor does it cover? What is the co-payment for these specialized services?

Chapter 6: References

1. "Affordable Care Act Tax Provisions," IRS. http://www.irs.gov/uac/Affordable-Care-Act-Tax-Provisions, accessed September 11, 2014. "Individual Mandate Fact Sheet," Blue Cross and Blue Shield. https://www.bcbsri.com/BCBSRIWeb/pdf/Individual_Mandate_Fact_Sheet.pdf, accessed September 11, 2014.

2. "Employer Health Benefits: 2014 Summary of Findings," Kaiser Family Foundation. http://files.kff.org/attachment/ehbs-2014-abstract-summary-of-findings, accessed May 25, 2015.

3. Jay MacDonald, "Health Insurance 'Sherpa'? Agent or Broker." Bankrate.com. http://www.bankrate.com/finance/insurance/health-insurance-sherpa-agent-or-broker-1.aspx, accessed May 25, 2015.

Chapter 7

OBAMACARE SUBSIDIES

Maryann O'Daniel was a self-employed writer living in Rhode Island. Her status as a business owner meant she could get health insurance on the private market before the ACA. However, after shopping around, the best deal she could get cost a whopping $842 a month, with a $5,000 deductible. That was the lowest rate she could find even though she was in good health. That's because she was 44 and lived in a high-cost state in New England. She paid at least $10,104 a year in premiums just to protect her health, her livelihood, and her life savings.

In October 2013, she researched plans on the Obamacare exchange and found one that cut her costs nearly in half. Her premium was just only $441 a month with a $2,500 deductible. This allowed her to invest more into her business and prepare for retirement.

Maryann also received an annual physical for free. She got her cholesterol, blood pressure, and blood sugar levels checked without spending hundreds of dollars. If there are ever any problems, she can work on getting them under control before they require an emergency room visit.

There are 25.7 million Americans like Maryann who are now eligible for federal subsidies that help them pay for health insurance. Nearly all of them (90 percent) have at least one family member who works. What types of jobs do they have? A study done for the State of Indiana by Families USA found they are employed as food service workers, administrative personnel, and health aides. They are also child-care workers, cashiers, and janitors. None of them make enough money to afford private health plans without help. Ron Pollack, executive director of Families USA, said, "It's not just for the poor. It reaches deeply into the middle class."[1]

You may be shocked to find out that the ACA will spend more on helping the middle class, like Maryann, than on the poor. More than half (56 percent) of the subsidies go to families who earn between $47,100 and $94,200 a year.

Subsidies for people who sign up on the exchanges will cost the federal government $1.039 trillion between 2015 and 2024. That's 30 percent more than the $792 billion being spent on expanded Medicaid and CHIP for the poor.[2]

Kaiser Health found that 60 percent of those who were eligible for Obamacare subsidies left money on the table. That means they could have gotten subsidies through the health-care exchanges in 2014, but didn't. How did Kaiser know that? There were seventeen million people who qualified for subsidies. These are people who:

- Did not have insurance from their employer.
- Made too much money to qualify for Medicaid.
- Were legal residents of the United States.

However, only 6.6 million *did* sign up. Are you one of the 10.4 million people who didn't?[3]

Who Really Benefits from the Subsidies?

The middle class is solidly in the crosshairs of Obamacare's subsidies. Anyone who makes 400 percent or less of the federal poverty level qualifies for a tax credit. (More on how this is calculated later in this chapter.) In 2015, that's $95,400 for a family of four.[4]

Surprised? A January 2014 Pew research survey found that only 44 percent of Americans report they are in the middle class. Almost as many (40 percent) say they are either lower-middle class or poor. And only 16 percent feel like they are upper-middle class or rich.

The Great Recession has a lot to do with this. In 2008, 53 percent of those surveyed said they were middle class. Only 25 percent said they were lower-middle class or poor, while 22 percent felt rich.

What happened? Obviously, a lot of people lost their jobs, homes, and retirement savings. However, people also *feel* less secure. That's true even if they earn the same amount as they did before the recession. Nearly 60 percent of people surveyed in the Country Financial Security Index are no longer sure that it's possible to live a middle-class existence in America *and* be financially secure.[5]

Part of the problem is that there's no official definition for middle-class income, as there is for poverty. People usually compare themselves to their friends, neighbors, or even try to keep up with the Kardashians.

There is, of course, national data on incomes. The most recent US census data tell us that the median income for a family of four is $79,698. That means half of the families this size make more, and half make less.

What if your household is smaller? The median income for a two-person family is $54,192, and for a three-person household it's $62,806.

Surprisingly, households with five or more people have a lower median income than those with just four members. That's because many high-income households have fewer children. In addition, families with more than two children usually require one parent to stay home and care for them. As a result, the median income for five-person households is $72,191; for six-person households is $67,247; and for seven-person households is $65,934.

How Obamacare Affects Four Different Income Groups

Just to give you an example of how Obamacare affects people by income, let's drill down into exactly how it affects these families of four. According to the statistics, 18 percent of American families of this size live on less than $32,913. They're all eligible for free health care from Medicaid.

The largest group are the 42 percent in the middle, who make between $32,913 and $94,200. These are the middle-income families who are eligible for subsidies.

Another 32 percent are in the upper-middle class, who make between $94,201 and $199,000. They don't receive subsidies but neither do they pay more in taxes.

The top 8 percent make $200,000 or more. They receive no subsidies, but must pay extra taxes.[6]

To keep things from getting too complicated, this example is just for families of four. To get a complete analysis, the same calculation could also be done for every family size and its income levels. You can still see from this example that the largest percentage (42 percent) are those in and around the median family income who are receiving subsidies. That's much greater than the 18 percent of families who are poor.

Understand How the Subsidies Work

To understand how the Obamacare subsidies work, you first need to understand how the federal poverty level (FPL) works. The FPL defines who the government considers to be living in poverty, based on income and family size. Like many other federal laws, the ACA uses the FPL as its basis in determining income eligibility for subsidies. Unlike many other laws, however, the ACA uses 2014 FPL to determine eligibility for 2015 subsidies, and the 2015 FPL to calculate eligibility for Medicaid and CHIP.

In 2014, the FPL started at $11,670 for a single-person household in the forty-eight contiguous states and the District of Columbia. The FPL was higher in two states where the cost of living is significantly higher: $13,420 in Hawaii and $14,580 in Alaska.

It added $4,060 for each additional person in the household ($4,670 in Hawaii and $5,080 in Alaska). It doesn't matter if those two people are a couple or a single parent with a child. So, if the two of you bring in $15,730 or less ($18,090 in Hawaii and $19,660 in Alaska), you're at the poverty level.

The federal breakdown for other family sizes:

- Three person = $19,790 ($22,760 in Hawaii and $24,740 in Alaska)
- Four person = $23,850 ($27,430 in Hawaii and $29,820 in Alaska)
- Five person = $27,910 ($32,100 in Hawaii and $34,900 in Alaska)
- Six person = $31,970 ($36,770 in Hawaii and $39,980 in Alaska)
- Seven person = $36,030 ($41,440 in Hawaii and $45,060 in Alaska)
- Eight person = $40,090 ($46,110 in Hawaii and $50,140 in Alaska)

In 2015, the FPL started at $11,770 for a single-person household in the forty-eight contiguous states and the District of Columbia. The 2015 FPL is $13,550 in Hawaii and $14,720 in Alaska.

It added $4,160 for each additional person ($4,780 on Hawaii and $5,200 in Alaska). The FPL for a two-person household is $15,930 ($18,330 in Hawaii and $19,920 in Alaska).

The federal breakdown for other family sizes:

- Three person = $20,090 ($23,110 in Hawaii and $25,120 in Alaska)
- Four person = $24,250 ($27,890 in Hawaii and $30,320 in Alaska)
- Five person = $28,410 ($32,670 in Hawaii and $35,520 in Alaska)
- Six person = $32,570 ($37,450 in Hawaii and $40,720 in Alaska)
- Seven person = $36,730 ($42,230 in Hawaii and $45,920 in Alaska)
- Eight person = $40,890 ($47,010 in Hawaii and $51,120 in Alaska)

The poverty level rises each year to keep up with inflation. HHS usually updates it in mid-January. You'll find it on the website at aspe.hhs.gov/poverty/index.cfm.

Five Levels of Subsidies

The ACA has five levels of subsidies. Each one is based on how much more you make than the poverty level. The higher your income, the lower the subsidy.

1. The first income bracket is 138 percent of the FPL. That means 38 percent more than the FPL. (The actual formula is FPL + 38 percent times FPL.)
2. 150 percent of the FPL.
3. 200 percent of the FPL, or two times the poverty level.
4. 250 of the FPL.
5. 400 percent of the FPL, or four times the poverty level.

Those who fall into the first income bracket qualify for Medicaid. However, your state had to agree to expand Medicaid, and twenty of them haven't as of 2015. All the other income levels receive a subsidy.

In addition, if your income is 225 percent of the poverty level or less, you can save more than most on your out-of-pocket costs for plans at the Silver level. Any insurance company that sells on the exchange must reduce these costs to an affordable level. For more, see www.healthcare.gov/choose-a-plan/out-of-pocket-costs/.

Subsidies Are Based on the Cost of the Silver Plan

The subsidy is not just a flat rate for everyone. Instead, the government bases it on the cost of a Silver plan in your area. (The four levels of insurance are explained in chapter 6.)

The subsidy is calculated to guarantee that you pay no more than 9.5 percent of your income for the second-lowest Silver plan. The subsidy will vary depending on your age, your income, your family size, and the cost of Silver plans in your state.

For example, a 38-year old couple earns the median income of $54,192. The cost of the second-lowest Silver plan in their area is $9,618 (also the national average).

The subsidy guarantees they won't pay more than 9.5 percent of their income for this plan. That's 0.95 times $54,192 which equals $5,148. The cost of the plan is $9,618. Their subsidy is $9,618 minus $5,148, or $4,469.

They can then apply the subsidy of $4,469 to any plan they want, either Bronze, Gold, or Platinum.[7]

The subsidy is automatically calculated on the healthcare.gov exchange. It also lets you choose whether you want your subsidy deducted from your premium each month or given directly to you at the end of the year as a tax break.

Are You Eligible for a Subsidy?

First, check to see if you are already receiving a subsidy. The Kaiser survey found that nearly half of those getting government subsidies through the exchanges don't even know they're getting anything. An official HHS report says 87 percent of those enrolled in the federal exchange are getting government subsidies but only 46 percent told Kaiser they were. That's probably because 43 percent said they found paying their premiums "difficult."[8]

Although most people complain that their premiums are too high, the CBO found that premiums under Obamacare were actually 16 percent lower than originally projected. And not only are the premiums lower, but more than 70 percent of individuals who buy through the exchanges also qualify for tax credits, making their premiums lower still. The US government estimates that six out of ten Americans who seek insurance through the exchanges will pay less than $100 a month for individual coverage.[9]

How close are you to the poverty level? That depends on how many people are in your household. The lower your household income, the more of an Obamacare tax credit you receive. You don't have to be at the poverty level to receive Obamacare subsidies. Even if your income is four times greater than the FPL, you'll still get something.

To see if you'll receive a subsidy, check the chart below. It shows the income level equivalent to 400 percent of the 2014 poverty level. If your household brings in less than this, then go to the exchanges to see if you can get a better deal on insurance than what you're currently getting:

- One person = $46,680
- Two person = $62,920
- Three person = $79,160
- Four person = $95,400
- Five person = $111,640
- Six person = $127,880
- Seven person = $144,120

- Eight person = $160,360

Here's an example. Let's say you're a family of four making $79,698 a year. You're using the exchange to find health insurance for yourself, your wife, and your two children. The 2014 poverty level for a family of four is $23,850. Four times that is $95,400, so you're within the 400 percent level. Now you know you'll receive a subsidy.

Determine Your Household Income

Many people are confused about what the IRS considers eligible household income. Basically, the size of your household and eligible income is based on anyone who is on your tax return and who needs insurance from the exchange.

First, figure out who is in your household. Make sure you include:

- You and your spouse, even if you normally file separate tax returns. That's because you will need to file jointly for the year you want subsidies. You must include your spouse's income, even if you only want insurance for yourself. However, if you are eligible for their job-based insurance, you may not be eligible for insurance on the exchanges or subsidies.
- Your children who live with you, even if they file their own tax returns.
- Anyone you list as a dependent on your tax return, even if they don't live with you.
- Anyone under twenty-one whom you take care of and who lives with you.
- Your unmarried partner *only* if they are your dependent for tax purposes or they are the parent of your child.

Don't include:

- Your unmarried partner's children if they are not your dependents.
- Your parents or other relatives who live with you, if they file their own tax return and aren't your dependents.
- Your children, if you and the other parent are divorced and you aren't claiming them as tax dependents.

Now that you know who's in your household, here's how to figure the income. For each person, add up wages, salaries, tips, net income from self-employment or business, unemployment compensation, Social Security payments, and alimony. To figure your wages, use the line on your pay stub that says "federal taxable wages." Don't forget to add retirement, investment and pension income, rental income, and income from prizes, awards, and gambling.

Don't include child support, gifts, Supplemental Security Income (SSI), veteran's disability payments, workers' comp, or money received from loans.[10]

Get Your Subsidy

The subsidy is added to your income tax refund. That's why if you don't file taxes, you can't receive a subsidy. The difference is that you don't have to wait until after you file your taxes to receive this refund. Most people tell the IRS to send the rebate directly to the insurance company each month to pay lower premiums. However, you can wait and get it as a rebate when you file your taxes.

If you wind up making a lot more than you reported, your subsidy could be reduced. If that happens, you might get hit with a larger tax bill at the end of the year. Therefore, make sure you update your account on the healthcare.gov website with any large income or household changes.

Chapter 7: References

1. Kelly Kennedy, "Study: Most Health Subsidies to Aid Working Families, *USA Today*, April 18, 2013. http://www.usatoday.com/story/news/nation/2013/04/18/states-exchange-subsidies/2090503/, accessed August 11, 2014. "Indiana Report: Working Individuals in Key Economic Sectors Make Up the Largest Group to Benefit by Extending Health Coverage," Families USA, August 6, 2014. http://familiesusa.org/press-release/2014/indiana-report-working-individuals-key-economic-sectors-make-largest-group, accessed August 11, 2014.

2. "Comparison of CBO's Estimates of the Net Budgetary Effects of the Coverage Provisions of the Affordable Care Act," Congressional Budget Office.

3. Kaiser Foundation, "Marketplace Enrollees Eligible for Financial Assistance as a Share of the Subsidy-Eligible Population," Kaiser Family Foundation, April 19, 2014. http://kff.org/health-reform/state-indicator/marketplace-enrollees-eligible-for-financial-assistance-as-a-share-of-the-subsidy-eligible-population/, accessed August 25, 2014.

4. Jared Bernstein, "The ACA Will Help, Not 'Frustrate,' the Middle Class," Huffington Post, December 22, 2013. http://www.huffingtonpost.com/jared-bernstein/obamacare-subsidies_b_4490575.html, accessed August 20, 2014.

5. Geoff Williams, "What It Means to Be Middle Class Today," *US News,* April 24, 2014. http://money.usnews.com/money/personal-finance/articles/2014/04/24/what-it-means-to-be-middle-class-today, accessed August 11, 2014.

6. Author's calculations based on "FINC-01. Selected Characteristics of Families by Total Money Income in 2012," *Current Population Survey, 2013 Annual Social and Economic Supplement,* US Census Bureau. http://www.census.gov/hhes/www/cpstables/032013/faminc/toc.htm, accessed August 11, 2014.

7. "Focus on Health Reform," Kaiser Family Foundation. http://kaiserfamilyfoundation.files.wordpress.com/2013/01/7962-02.pdf, accessed August 20, 2014.

8. "Survey Says: ObamaCare Isn't Doing So Well," Investor's Business Daily, June 24, 2014. http://news.investors.com/ibd-editorials-obama-care/062414-706031-kaiser-obamacare-survey-is-nothing-to-cheer-about-webhed-survey-says-obamacare-isnt-doing-so-well.htm, accessed August 12, 2014.

9. Ellen Goldbaum, "Who Will the Affordable Care Act Benefit the Most?" University at Buffalo, October 1, 2013. http://www.buffalo.edu/news/releases/2013/10/002.html, accessed August 30, 2014.

10. "What's Included as Income," Healthcare.gov. https://www.healthcare.gov/income-and-household-information/income/, accessed Mary 25, 2015.

Chapter 8

MANDATORY COVERAGE LOWERS COSTS

Usually, people only think about getting insurance when they start having children, have an accident or become ill themselves, or notice their friends succumbing to disease. In other words, they only buy insurance when they need it. As explained in chapter 4, insurance is profitable only when companies can spread the risk among a large group of people who mostly don't need it. To make premiums lower for everyone, the ACA mandates that even healthy people must either get insured or pay a tax. As this requirement kicks in, it will lower costs for insurance companies, who will pass those savings on to everyone.

The mandate allows the ACA to ban preexisting condition clauses. Most people don't understand that the two must go hand-in-hand. Otherwise, everyone would just wait until they got sick before applying for insurance. That would be like applying for car insurance after your accident.

The system would no longer be insurance; it would be government-provided health care. That's because no health insurance company could stay in business if it didn't receive premiums from healthy people.

The only reason that insurance worked until now is because company-sponsored insurance does spread that risk among all workers. However, even employer-sponsored insurance coverage fell 10 percent in the decade prior to the ACA. That means 4.5 million workers lost their company-sponsored health plans and had to find coverage on their own. Employers also cut their share of contributing to benefits. That means even those workers who kept their plans paid more and more for the very same plan. For them, insurance costs started rising in 1999.

Before 2010, private, non-company plans only covered twelve million people. Private plans either cost more than company plans or provided less coverage. Most did both. They denied you if you had a preexisting condition like arthritis, back pain, or a diagnosis that even remotely sounded like cancer. They could cancel your plan after you got sick. If you had a heart attack, the insurance company could drop you and you literally could not get insured again. Plans had lifetime limits. Once your illness cost more than, say, $2 million, they wouldn't pay any more. You'd either have to find the money yourself or just not get treated.

Some states tried to make these practices illegal. They required insurance companies to cover anyone and everyone. Sick people came out of the woodwork. Others just waited until they got sick and then bought insurance. That's like waiting until after your car gets totaled before buying insurance. Insurers quit offering plans in those states. Others doubled their premiums to cover the cost of all these suddenly insured sick people.

The best way to solve the problem was to mandate that everyone get insurance. That means the insurance companies would receive premiums from healthy people who didn't cost them much. That would pay for the cost of the sick people's treatment.

This doesn't really seem fair, does it? Why should healthy people be forced to pay for insurance they probably don't need?

It's just like car insurance, homeowners insurance, or even renters insurance. You pay premiums month after month, and consider yourself lucky if you don't need it. You are essentially paying the insurance company for all others who get in accidents or have their houses burn down. However, it's worth it to you because you can't afford to lose your car or your home. You can't afford to have your life savings wiped out by one bad event.

Health insurance works exactly the same way. Your chances of having a heart attack, getting cancer, or needing treatment for diabetes is much higher than that of having your house burn down or totaling your car. That's all insurance is—paying a monthly fee in exchange for someone else paying for a devastating event.

To make insurance work for the companies, you can't allow people to only sign up when they need it. To make it work for people, you can't allow companies to cancel coverage after they become sick or if they have a preexisting condition. There are only three ways around this, and the best one right now is mandatory insurance. The other two are: no insurance at all (letting everyone find their own way to pay for health care) or having the government provide it to everyone (like public education).

Of course, if there's a mandate, it's not fair to force people to pay for insurance they can't afford. Some people are barely making ends meet and are living paycheck to paycheck. That's why, if there's a mandate, there must also be a subsidy.

That's the three-legged stool that made health insurance reform work in Massachusetts under Governor Mitt Romney. And that's the plan that, ironically, Obamacare is modeled after.[1]

What the Mandate Actually Says

The mandate requires everyone in America to either have health insurance or pay a higher tax. In reality, everyone in America will instead fall into one of the following four categories:

Ineligible for Obamacare and exempt from the tax. You must fulfill certain requirements to even be eligible for Obamacare. If you fall into one of these categories and aren't eligible, then you won't have to pay a tax even if you don't get insurance.

- You have to be a legal US resident That means, contrary to popular opinion, the eleven million illegal immigrants cannot get either Obamacare or Medicaid legally. They can go to community health clinics where they pay on a sliding-fee basis. (Note: Everyone, including illegal immigrants, is covered by Medicaid for emergency room treatment only if they otherwise can't afford it.)
- You can't be in jail. Health care for the 2.5 million U.S. prisoners is provided by the penal system.

Eligible for Obamacare but exempt from the tax. By 2016, there will be twenty-six million people who will remain uninsured even though they are eligible for Obamacare insurance. That's 87 percent of the uninsured, and they don't have to pay the tax.[2]

That's because they have successfully filed for an exemption. For example, they didn't make enough to pay income taxes, or their premiums were more than 8.05 percent of their income. To see if you qualify for an exemption, see chapter 6.[3]

Have qualifying insurance. There are 250 million people who already have insurance that qualifies under the ACA. Many people lost their insurance plans in 2014 because their plans didn't comply with the ACA's requirements. The following types of health insurance did comply:

- Medicare, Medicaid, CHIP, TRICARE, or the Veterans Administration.
- Your employer's health plan.
- A private health plan that covers the ten essential benefits.
- A private health plan that was in existence before 2010 and has been grandfathered in.
- Catastrophic insurance if you are under age thirty or qualify for a "hardship exemption."
- Health insurance purchased on the Obamacare exchange.
- Your parents' health plan if you are under age twenty-six.[4]

Pay the tax. Anyone who doesn't fall into one of the above categories will be required to pay an additional income tax. The tax penalty doubles to 2 percent of your income in 2015 (no less than $325) and 2.5 percent in 2016 (at least $695). See chapter 10 for a detailed description of the tax rates.

It's estimated that four million people, or only 13 percent of the uninsured, fall into this category. That's because so many people either aren't eligible for Obamacare or are exempt. [5]

Will the Mandate Work?

Without the mandate, insurance companies cannot afford to both offer universal coverage and reduce costs. The goal of the individual mandate is to get enough uninsured, healthy people to pay for the newly insured sick people. That percentage should be 40 percent healthy to 60 percent unhealthy. Since the data collected doesn't really show who is healthy versus who is sick, the goal is to have that ratio be young people to older ones.

What happens if enough young people don't sign up? The total premiums collected by insurers won't be enough. That's because the income from premiums must cover health-care claims plus the insurers' cost of doing business plus profit. If that's the case, insurance companies will probably raise premiums to stay in business.[6]

Eight million people signed up on the health-care exchanges during the 2014 enrollment period. Of those, 28 percent were between 18 and 34. Although this is lower than the 40 percent goal, the CBO estimates that the number of enrollees will rise to 12 million in calendar year 2015 and quadruple to 27 million by 2017. That's such a large increase that it's too soon to say what the final ratio of young-to-old enrollees will be.[7]

The Mandate and Medicaid

One way to make sure enough healthy people sign up is to expand Medicaid. Before Obamacare, single adults without children weren't eligible for Medicaid at all. The expanded Medicaid program is now available for those adults, and the so-called working poor, whose income falls under 138 percent of the poverty level. That's $16,243 for singles and $33,465 for a family of four. Go to chapter 7 for more on how these levels work.

The expansion does two things. Of course, it allows more people to get health insurance. This could raise costs of Obamacare initially because more people will discover previously ignored illnesses and seek treatment. It also allows people without other resources to get preventive care and avoid expensive emergency room visits.

However, nearly half the states did not agree to expand Medicaid coverage, even though the federal government was footing most of the bill. States said they couldn't even afford the portion they would pay, while others said Medicaid didn't really work. It may be a coincidence that every state that didn't expand it was led by the Republican Party.

That means the people in those states could not take advantage of government-sponsored health insurance. If they could afford it, they could still go on the exchanges and get subsidies for health insurance. They also have community health centers, paid for by Obamacare, that are open to everyone.

Even in the states that didn't expand Medicaid coverage, people started coming out of the woodwork to apply for non-expanded Medicaid. Just over half a million signed up during the first enrollment period (October 2013 to March 2014). These were people who qualified for Medicaid even before the ACA, but had never bothered to sign up for whatever reason.[8]

Many people signed up simply to avoid the penalty, while others responded to massive outreach efforts. The benefit is that these people can now get preventive care, which should reduce the number of emergency room visits. It should lower health-care costs even for those states that opposed Obamacare.

Chapter 8: References

1. "Why the Individual Mandate is Effective and Efficient," The Daily Beast, March 26, 2012. http://www.thedailybeast.com/articles/2012/03/26/why-the-individual-mandate-is-effective-and-efficient.html, accessed October 26, 2014.

2. Jo Craven McGinty, "How the Tally of Illegal Immigrants Adds Up," *The Wall Street Journal*, March 13, 2015. http://www.wsj.com/articles/how-the-tally-of-illegal-immigrants-adds-up-and-why-it-matters-1426259113, accessed July 9, 2015. "America's Prison Population," *The Economist*, March 13, 2014. http://www.economist.com/blogs/democracyinamerica/2014/03/americas-prison-population, accessed July 9, 2015. "Payments of Penalties for Being Uninsured Under the Affordable Care Act: 2014 Update," Congressional Budget Office, June 5, 2014. http://www.cbo.gov/publication/45397, accessed October 26, 2014.

3. "Hardship Exemptions From the Fee for Not Having Health Insurance," HealthCare.gov. https://www.healthcare.gov/fees-exemptions/exemptions-from-the-fee/, accessed October 26, 2014.

4. Joanne Kenen, "5 Myths of the Individual Mandate," Politico, June 28, 2012. http://www.politico.com/news/stories/0612/77997.html, accessed October 26, 2014.

5. "Payments of Penalties," Congressional Budget Office.

6. Larry Levitt, Gary Claxton, and Anthony Damico, "The Numbers Behind 'Young Invincibles' and the Affordable Care Act," Kaiser Family Foundation, December 17, 2013. http://kff.org/health-reform/perspective/the-numbers-behind-young-invincibles-and-the-affordable-care-act/, accessed October 26, 2014.

7. "Health Insurance Marketplace: Summary Enrollment Report," ASPE Issue Brief. http://aspe.hhs.gov/health/reports/2014/marketplaceenrollment/apr2014/ib_2014apr_enrollment.pdf, accessed October 26, 2014. "Insurance Coverage Provisions of the Affordable Care Act-CBO March 2015 Baseline, Table 3," Congressional Budget Office, March 2015. https://www.cbo.gov/sites/default/files/cbofiles/attachments/43900-2015-03-ACAtables.pdf, accessed June 18, 2015.

8. Jason Millman, "These States Rejected Medicaid Expansion, But Medicaid Is Expanding Anyway," *Washington Post*, May 13, 2014. http://www.washingtonpost.com/blogs/wonkblog/wp/2014/05/13/these-states-rejected-obamacares-medicaid-expansion-but-medicaid-is-expanding-there-anyway/, accessed October 26, 2014.

Chapter 9

WHO ELSE BENEFITS?

Many people don't realize how much Obamacare benefits seniors, small business owners, and even charities. That's because the benefits it confers on Medicare, as discussed in chapter 3, aren't well publicized by the media. Remember, the primary purpose of the ACA is to lower the cost of health care, Medicare, and Medicaid. Anything that lowers those costs helps seniors, most of whom are on Medicare, and many of whom are also on Medicaid.

Seniors

The ACA made many changes that benefit everyone on Medicare, most of whom are seniors 65 years of age or older. Below is the income breakdown of Medicare recipients:

- **Low income (35 percent).** 17 percent are below the poverty level, while another 18 percent are between 100 and 140 percent of the poverty level. Most, therefore, qualify for Medicaid, which was raised to 138 percent of the poverty level by the ACA.
- **Middle income (34 percent).** 13 percent are between 150 and 200 percent of the poverty level. Another 21 percent are between 201 and 300 percent of the poverty level.
- **Upper-middle income and high income (31 percent).** 31 percent earn more than 300 percent of the poverty level.[1]

The ACA requires Medicare to extend free preventive care to its beneficiaries.

It also eliminates the donut hole in Medicare Part D Prescription Drug benefits. Before the ACA, Medicare paid 75 percent of the first $2,800 (in 2010) in prescription drug costs once the patient reached the $310 deductible. Then the patient fell into the donut hole and had to pay 100 percent of drug costs up to $4,550 (again, in 2010). That's when Medicare coverage kicked in again, paying 95 percent of drug costs.

The ACA required Medicare Part D insurance plans to pay 50 percent of the donut hole costs in 2011, rising to 75 percent in 2020. In 2015, the coverage gap began at $2,960, rising to $3,310 in 2016. At that point, you pay 45 percent for brand-name drugs, and 65 percent for generic drugs. Drug companies are being charged higher fees to help cover this subsidy. As of 2015, at least 8.2 million seniors are saving $11.5 billion.[2]

Obamacare also fights Medicare fraud, which will lower the cost to seniors. It gives fraud fighters these new tools:

Tougher sentences for criminals. The ACA increases federal sentencing guidelines by 20 to 50 percent for fraud that cost more than $1 million in damages.

Enhanced screening. Requires high-risk providers and suppliers to undergo more scrutiny, such as license checks and site visits.

State-of-the-art technology. CMS will be able to take advantage of advanced predictive modeling technology to screen for fraudulent activity.

New resources. The law provides an additional $350 million in funding.[2]

Additionally, the ACA reduces payments to Medicare Advantage plans, which had been overcharging the government. As a result of all these measures, the government has gotten back a record-breaking $10.7 billion in recoveries of health-care fraud in the last three years.[3]

Small Businesses and Charities

Small businesses (companies with fifty or fewer employees) make up 96 percent of the six million businesses in the United States. They are critical for reducing unemployment among the middle class, since they are responsible for creating 65 percent of all new jobs. Small business owners are in the middle class, with only 3 percent earning $250,000 a year or more.

The Affordable Care Act set aside $37 billion to help small businesses provide health insurance. First, federal financial assistance is available to small businesses that offer health insurance to early retirees, age fifty-five to sixty-four. Second, companies receive a 50 percent tax credit on premiums they pay for their employees. Tax-exempt businesses and charities get a 35 percent tax credit.[4]

Chapter 9: References

1. "The Medicare Beneficiary Population," AARP Public Policy Institute. http://assets. aarp.org/rgcenter/health/fs149_medicare.pdf, accessed November 4, 2014.
2. Jonathan Blum, "What Is the Donut Hole?" The Medicare Blog, August 9, 2010. http:// blog.medicare.gov/2010/08/09/what-is-the-donut%C2%A0hole/, accessed October 6, 2014. "Costs in the Coverage Gap," Medicare.gov. http://www.medicare.gov/part-d/ costs/coverage-gap/part-d-coverage-gap.html, accessed June 18, 2015. "Closing the Donut Hole," National Committee to Preserve Social Security and Medicare. http:// www.ncpssm.org/Medicare/ClosingtheDonutHole, accessed June 18, 2015.
3. "The Affordable Care Act and Fighting Fraud," Stop Medicare Fraud. http://www.stop medicarefraud.gov/aboutfraud/aca-fraud/index.html, accessed October 6, 2014.
4. "Small Business Health Care Tax Credit and the SHOP Marketplace," IRS. http:// www.irs.gov/uac/Small-Business-Health-Care-Tax-Credit-and-the-SHOP-Market place, accessed May 26, 2015.

Chapter 10

WHO PAYS FOR OBAMACARE?

The idea that Obamacare is a wealth redistribution program that taxes the middle class and rewards the poor is not entirely true. Here's a look at exactly who pays and how much.

The ACA is paid for in three ways: reduced payments to providers, tax increases on higher income households and many businesses, and higher fees to some health-care providers and cost savings in programs. Below is a description of each and an estimate for an average year (2019). By then, all of the changes will be fully operational.

Health-Care Providers

The ACA allows the federal government to reduce Medicare and Medicaid payments to health-care providers. That's a critical first step to reduce the skyrocketing cost of Medicare, the third largest item in the federal budget (after Social Security and all defense spending). For more details on the budget, see chapter 2.

This cost savings is the largest source of funding, totaling $94 billion in 2019. Hospitals, doctors' offices, and drug companies are willing to accept these reduced payments in return for the larger number of insured patients that Obamacare will bring in. Here are the four major categories of reductions:

Reduced Medicare payments ($53 billion). Every year, Medicare agrees on certain payment rates for covered services to health-care providers. These annual updates are reduced by 21 percent. Hospital groups expect to more than make up the loss by treating fewer uninsured patients. The rest will come from skilled nursing facilities and home health agencies.

Reduced Medicare Advantage overpayments ($18 billion). These private health plans cover one in five seniors. Medicare pays Medicare Advantage insurance companies over 14 percent more than is spent per person in traditional Medicare. This results in increased premiums for all Medicare beneficiaries, including the 69 percent of beneficiaries who are not currently enrolled in a Medicare Advantage plan. The law levels the playing field by gradually eliminating this discrepancy. People enrolled in a Medicare Advantage plan will still receive all guaranteed Medicare benefits, and the law provides bonus payments to Medicare Advantage plans that provide high quality care. Savings started in 2011.

Reduced Medicare and Medicaid DSH payments ($10 billion). Some hospitals are located in areas with many low-income people who use the emergency room as their primary care provider. As a result, these hospitals use a disproportionate share (DSH) of their budgets to pay for these services. To compensate, Medicare and Medicaid pay these hospitals extra. Hospitals were willing to take a cut in these payments since expanded Medicaid and community health centers should result in fewer emergency room visits.

Other provisions ($13 billion). This category contains many small savings that will be made to Medicare, Medicaid, and CHIP. For example, some of the savings come from more efficient spending on prescription drugs and biologics. Others arise from suggestions made by the Independent Payment Advisory Board (IPAB). A third saving is from lower prescription drug subsidies for seniors who earn at least $85,000 a year (or married couples who earn $170,000).

Families

New taxes are the second-largest source of funds, bringing in $92 billion in 2019. The largest amount ($66.7 billion) comes from families. Here's exactly who's affected:

High-income family tax ($38 billion). Income and capital gains taxes were increased for five million high-income families in 2013. That's one million individuals who make more than $200,000 a year, and four million married couples who make more than $250,000 annually. This income threshold is based on Adjusted Gross Income.[1]

There are two taxes that apply. The first is an additional 0.9 percent Medicare hospital tax on income and self-employment profits above the threshold. It raises the tax from 2.9 percent to 3.8 percent. If you're self-employed, you pay the total 3.8 percent tax. Otherwise, you pay 2.35 percent while your employer pays the remaining 1.45 percent as it has always done.

How much is that? For a person making $300,000 a year, the extra tax is around $9,000. If that sounds like a lot to you, remember that to someone at that income level, it's the cost of a Birkin purse.

The second tax is an extra 3.8 percent on any investment income earned by people whose AGI is above the threshold described above. This income includes common interest, dividends, and capital gains. It also includes rental and royalty income, non-qualified annuities, income from businesses that trade securities or commodities, and businesses that are passive activities.[2]

This capital gains tax only applies to profits from selling the home you live in when certain conditions are met. First, your AGI must be more than the threshold. Second, the profit from selling your home must be more than $250,000 (singles) or $500,000 (married couples). Keep in mind, that's not the sale price of your home; that's the amount you've cleared above and beyond what you've spent on your home. This threshold only applies to your home, not to investment property, which is treated like any other capital gains. Third, the 3.8 percent tax is only applied to the amount above the threshold.[3]

Employees who receive higher wages in lieu of employer insurance ($16 billion). The Congressional Budget Office (CBO) estimates 16 million employees will not be offered, or won't take, health insurance benefits from their employer. Instead, the CBO assumes many of those companies will pay higher wages, in lieu of the benefits, to retain valued employees.

Health insurance isn't taxable, but higher wages are. As a result, these higher wages will generate more federal income tax revenue. Of course, that assumes the businesses don't simply pocket the "extra wages" instead of giving them to employees.

The CBO assumes that workers will have enough power to demand, and get, higher wages instead of health benefits. This hasn't been the experience of most workers since the recession. Therefore, this $16 billion income estimate may not actually materialize.

Other tax changes ($7.7 billion). There are many other tax changes that generate smaller amounts of revenue. Here are just four of them.

First, if you have high medical costs that aren't covered by insurance, you were able to deduct all costs that were above 7.5 percent of your AGI. Now you can only deduct the costs that are above 10 percent of your AGI.

Second, you can only put $2,500 of pretax income into a tax-deferred Flexible Spending Account. However, you can transfer $500 of any unused funds into the next year. Before the ACA, there was no limit on how much you could put in, but you had to use all the funds or lose them.[4]

Third, if you withdraw money from a health savings account for non-medical expenses before age sixty-five, you pay a 20 percent penalty instead of a 10 percent penalty.

Fourth, you are no longer able to use these accounts to buy over-the-counter medicines for allergy relief and similar items without a doctor's prescription (there's an exception for insulin).

Those without insurance ($5 billion). The smallest contribution is from the uninsured. You must be insured for at least nine months out of the year or pay an additional income tax. The CBO and JCT (Joint Committee on Taxation) estimate that four million people will be without insurance and pay the tax.

Businesses

The contribution from businesses that aren't health-care providers is $25.3 billion. There are three main taxes:

Employer penalties ($15 billion). Companies with 50 or more full-time equivalent employees (FTE) that don't offer insurance pay an excise tax of $2,000 per employee, except for the first thirty employees. This tax also applies to companies that offer plans that don't meet the ACA standards. In addition, plans must cost no more than 9.5 percent of the employee's income, and pay for at least 60 percent of covered benefits. Companies with fewer than 100 FTEs that certify they haven't intentionally made reductions or laid off workers to avoid the penalties can get the tax waived.[5]

Companies that offer Cadillac plans ($10 billion). Companies pay a 40 percent excise tax on the Cadillac plan premiums (the tax starts in 2018). These are high-end health insurance policies with annual premiums of at least $10,200 (individuals) or $27,500 (families). They are typically offered for three reasons:

1. They provide extra coverage for those in dangerous jobs.
2. They are offered by companies that have an unusual number of chronically ill or elderly employees.
3. They offer extra benefits to high-level employees.

Dental and vision plans are exempt and will not be counted in the total cost of a family's plan.[6]

Indoor tanning services ($0.3 billion). In 2010, these companies were hit with an excise tax of 10 percent of the actual cost of tanning. About 80 percent said they passed the cost along to their customers. Why tanners? Because the radiation is a source for skin cancer. However, the price hike didn't really hurt their business, with only one in four saying they saw a decline in revenue after the tax was passed.[7]

Health Insurance Companies

The smallest revenue category consists of extra fees imposed on some health-care providers. That will contribute $40 billion in 2019, our sample year.

Additional fees on health insurance companies, prescription drug makers, and importers ($18 billion). In 2013, companies like Medtronic started paying an additional 2.3 percent excise tax on gross sales. Some retail products are excluded, such as glasses, contact lens, and hearing aids. The drug and health insurance companies agreed to these additional fees because the cost will be more than outweighed by additional revenues from the new customers that are being insured.[8]

Reinsurance and risk adjustment ($22 billion). This is a new program that makes sure some insurance companies don't get penalized by the changes in the ACA. It spreads the risk around to the entire industry. Insurance companies will pay into a pool, and those companies with a higher-than-average group of sick enrollees will receive a refund to help pay for the costs. The taxes collected will cover the cost of the program, so you'll see it in both taxes and benefits.

It's actually three separate programs created by Obamacare for health insurers.

1. Reinsurance transfers funds from group health plans, which have lower risk, to private health plans, which have greater risks. This transfer is only from 2014 through 2016 since it's a temporary program designed to make the transition smoother.
2. Risk corridor limits issuers' losses and gains. It's for all health plans and also lasts from 2014 through 2016.
3. Risk adjustment transfers funds from low-risk to high risk private health plans. It has no time limit.[9]

Who Pays the Most?

You may have heard that the ACA will impose an additional $1 trillion in tax hikes, aimed squarely at middle-income families. It is true that it adds at least $1 trillion in taxes over a ten-year period (2013 to 2022). Most of the taxes don't affect families, however. Here's how it actually breaks down.

Big business pays the most taxes, around $350 billion. Here's the businesses that are taxed:

- The biggest amount is paid by prescription drug companies, like Pfizer, and medical device makers, like Medtronic. They'll pay a 2.3 percent excise tax on sales, totaling $180 billion by 2022. However, they also receive more customers from the health insurance mandate.
- Indoor tanning services pay $3 billion in additional taxes over ten years.
- Starting in 2015, companies with 50 or more employees who don't provide insurance will pay $130 billion in penalty taxes, according to the CBO.
- Starting in 2018, companies that offer Cadillac plans will contribute $40 billion from a 40 percent excise tax.

Families making $200,000 or more will pay a third of the total tax bill. That's $318 billion paid through increased payroll and investment taxes, starting in 2013.

Middle income families will pay the remaining third. A total of $377 billion in direct and indirect taxes will roll out between 2013 and 2022. Below are five ways the ACA taxes everyone:

1. Fewer medical expenses can be deducted from your taxes. Before the ACA, you could deduct any costs that were above 7.5 percent of your AGI. Now your medical expenses must be more than 10 percent of your AGI.
2. Only $2,500 of pretax income can be put into a tax-deferred Flexible Spending Account (FSA). Before, the amount was unlimited.[10]
3. The penalty you pay on money you withdraw from a health savings account for non-medical expenses before age 65 has doubled—from 10 percent to 20 percent.
4. FSAs can no longer be used to buy over-the-counter medicines (except insulin) without a prescription.
5. Taxes will be owed to the IRS if you aren't covered by health insurance for nine months of the year.

However, as you've learned in this book, the middle-class families receive far more in subsidies than they pay out in taxes. The CBO calculates they get a total of $1 trillion in premium credits in the same ten-year period—more than double what they pay in taxes. On a net basis, they come out ahead.[11]

Chapter 10: References

1. "Medicare Advantage," Kaiser Family Foundation, June 29, 2015. Ryan Donmoyer, "Obama Spreads the Wealth," Bloomberg, March 22, 2010.

2. "Questions and Answers on the Net Investment Tax," IRS. http://www.irs.gov/uac/Newsroom/Net-Investment-Income-Tax-FAQs, accessed September 9, 2014.

3. Tara-Nicholle Nelson, "Demystifying Obamacare Real Estate Tax," Inman News, February 14, 2013. http://www.inman.com/2013/02/14/demystifying-obamacare-real-estate-tax/, accessed September 11, 2014.

4. "Treasury Modifies Use-or-Lose Rule for Health Spending Accounts," US Treasury, October 31, 2013. http://www.treasury.gov/press-center/press-releases/Pages/jl2202.aspx, accessed September 11, 2014.

5. Jean Murray, "How Obamacare Affects Small Businesses," About.com. http://biztaxlaw.about.com/od/healthcarebusinesstax/f/How-Does-Health-Care-Law-Affect-Business.htm, accessed September 11, 2014. Josh Hicks, "Obamacare Tax Hikes vs. Tax Breaks: Which Is Greater?" *Washington Post* Factchecker, July 6, 2012. http://www.washingtonpost.com/blogs/fact-checker/post/obamacare-tax-hikes-vs-tax-breaks-which-is-greater/2012/07/06/gJQAx6AyPW_blog.html, accessed September 11, 2014.

6. Jenny Gold, "Cadillac Insurance Plans Explained," Kaiser Health News, March 18, 2010. http://kaiserhealthnews.org/news/cadillac-tax-explainer-update/, accessed September 11, 2014. William Perez, "Tax Impacts of the Supreme Court's Decision," About.com. http://taxes.about.com/b/2012/07/03/tax-impacts-of-the-supreme-courts-health-care-decision.htm, accessed September 11, 2014.

7. Andrew M. Seaman, "U.S. Indoor Tanning Tax Having Mixed Effects," Reuters, January 19, 2012. http://www.reuters.com/article/2012/01/19/us-ndoor-tanning-idUSTRE80I25V20120119, accessed September 11, 2014.

8. "Medical Device Tax," IRS. http://www.irs.gov/uac/Newsroom/Medical-Device-Excise-Tax, accessed September 11, 2014.

9. Author's calculations based on the following sources: "Reinsurance, Risk Corridors, and Risk Adjustment Final Rule," Center for Medicare and Medicaid Services, March 2012. http://www.cms.gov/cciio/resources/files/downloads/3rs-final-rule.pdf, accessed September 11, 2014. "Letter to Honorable Nancy Pelosi," Congressional

Budget Office and Joint Committee on Taxation, March 20, 2010, Table 2. http://www.cbo.gov/sites/default/files/cbofiles/ftpdocs/113xx/doc11379/amendreconprop.pdf, accessed September 9, 2014. "Updated Estimates of the Effects of the Insurance Coverage Provisions of the ACA," Congressional Budget Office, March 2012. http://cbo.gov/sites/default/files/cbofiles/attachments/03-13-Coverage%20Estimates.pdf, accessed September 9, 2014. "Letter to Honorable John Boehner," Congressional Budget Office and Joint Committee on Taxation, July 24, 2012. http://www.cbo.gov/sites/default/files/cbofiles/attachments/43471-hr6079.pdf, accessed September 9, 2014. "Updated Estimates of the Effects of the Insurance Coverage Provisions of the ACA," Congressional Budget Office, April 2014. http://cbo.gov/sites/default/files/cbofiles/attachments/45231-ACA_Estimates.pdf, accessed September 9, 2014.

10. "Treasury Modifies Use-or-Lose Rule for Health Spending Accounts," US Treasury, October 31, 2013. http://www.treasury.gov/press-center/press-releases/Pages/jl2202.aspx, accessed September 4, 2014.

11. Glenn Kess, "Does 'Obamacare' Have $1 Trillion in Tax Hikes, Aimed at the Middle Class?" *Washington Post*, March 12, 2103. http://www.washingtonpost.com/blogs/fact-checker/post/does-obamacare-have-1-trillion-in-tax-hikes-aimed-at-the-middle-class/2013/03/11/1e685f4c-8a9b-11e2-8d72-dc76641cb8d4_blog.html, accessed August 25, 2014.

CONCLUSION

Congratulations! You took the time to not just survive Obamacare but learn how to thrive by it. You now have the power to join the 100 million Americans who have benefited from the Affordable Care Act. You're armed with the knowledge to make your own decisions based on how the law affects you and the people you care about the most.

You've gotten the research-based facts that show how the ACA is not only making health care available to more middle-class families, but also, more importantly, modernizing health care and therefore lowering costs for everyone. You've also read true stories of real people who have been helped by the ACA.

You can return to this handbook again and again in case you want to review the basics. You can explain to your friends how health insurance works. You can use the step-by-step guides to sign up for insurance using the online exchanges. You can refer to the bonus sections at the end of this book that define key phrases, and impress your friends at parties by your in-depth knowledge of arcane medical terms!

Most importantly, you're now able to read between the lines of the controversial news articles, since you understand all the terms used. You also know the players—the authors of the ACA, the hospitals that were involved in the pilot programs, the large insurance companies that profited, the federal agencies that manage it all—and what their agendas are. You'll have the facts to back up your opinions.

You now know that the most important objective of Obamacare is *already* being achieved—lower costs of health care. This helps everyone. That includes our parents, grandparents, and most importantly our children, who have to foot the bill for future Medicare costs.

HOW TO SPEAK OBAMACARE: KEY WORDS AND PHRASES YOU NEED TO KNOW

ACA (Affordable Care Act): The full name is the Patient Protection and Affordable Care Act of 2010. This 2,572-page document was signed into law on March 23, 2010. It significantly changed health care in the United States. It's also known as Obamacare after President Barack Obama.

ACO (Accountable Care Organization): Affiliated hospitals, clinics, and medical practices agree to work together to focus on your health care. This improves your care and lowers costs. Your primary care doctor works with her hospital and its specialists, pharmacists, and nurses to coordinate care. To do this, they share an integrated electronic health record system. They also share any cost savings with Medicare. Ultimately, this will be expanded to health insurance companies and their beneficiaries, not just Medicare.

Activities of Daily Living (ADL): These are everyday tasks that a healthy person should be able to do by themselves to live independently. A person can lose the ability to do these tasks through disability, an accident, disease, or just by general old age. When this happens, they generally require assistance, either in the home or at a facility. The most often used measure is the Katz Activities of Daily Living. There are six: eating, bathing, dressing, transferring (from bed to standing, for example), using the toilet, and continence.

AGI (Adjusted Gross Income): According to the IRS, your Adjusted Gross Income is gross income minus adjustments to income. These adjustments include things like alimony payments, contributions to retirement accounts like a traditional IRA, and deductions for tuition. For the self-employed, it includes half of the self-employment taxes. It doesn't include exemptions or deductions, whether standard or itemized. For that reason, it's a bigger number than your taxable income. It is indicated on your federal income tax return: Line 4 on Form 1040EZ, Line 21 on Form 1040A, or Line 37 on Form 1040.

Ambulatory Surgery Center: Outpatient centers that perform minor surgeries, whether to correct a disease or diagnose a condition. They provide same-day surgery, are designed for simple procedures, and are a convenient alternative to traditional hospitals. According to the Ambulatory Surgery Center Association, common specialties include plastic surgery, eye surgery, orthopedics, and procedures to manage or eliminate pain.

Annual Cap: Insurance companies used to pay up to an annual limit, usually one or two million dollars. After the limit, you were responsible for the rest. This has been banned under the ACA.

Assisted Living Facility: Provides help with the activities of daily living. Requires special insurance for assisted living. It's not covered by regular health insurance or Medicare, which typically only cover three days of skilled nursing facility care.

Automatic Enrollment: The ACA requires companies with more than two hundred full-time employees to automatically enroll new employees into a health-care plan. The worker can always opt out.

Bronze Plan: The insurance pays 60 percent of your health-care costs, while you pay 40 percent overall. You can choose the mixture of deductibles, co-pays, and coinsurance.

Cadillac Plan: These are usually employer plans that have premiums of at least $10,200 (individuals) or $27,500 (families) per year. They're called Cadillac because they offer exceptional coverage. They are typically offered for those with high health needs. Many are required because the employees work in a dangerous occupation. Other companies may find the majority of its employees have chronic diseases, are older, or live in an area with expensive health costs. They are also used to offer extra benefits to high-level employees. For more, go to www.

kaiserhealthnews.org/stories/2009/september/22/cadillac-health-explainer-npr. aspx.

Capitation: The doctor receives a fixed amount per month per patient from a managed care plan instead of being paid for each test or procedure (see fee-for-service). The doctor profits by being more efficient.

Catastrophic Health Insurance: It usually only covers hospitalization and has a lower premium as a result. These plans are no longer available under the ACA unless you are under thirty or qualify for a hardship exemption. Catastrophic plans available to those groups have high deductibles but do pay for essential health benefits once the deductible is reached. They also offer free preventive care.

CHIP: The Children's Health Insurance Program was established in 1997. It covers eight million children aged nineteen and younger in families with incomes too high to qualify for Medicaid, but too low to get private health insurance. The federal government provides matching funds and the states manage it. In most programs, children and teens receive free or low-cost regular checkups, shots, doctor and dentist visits, vision care, hospital care, mental health services, and required prescriptions. Cost is based on the parents' income.

CMS (Centers for Medicare and Medicaid Services): The department of HHS that manages Medicare, Medicaid, and Obamacare.

Coinsurance: This is the percent of each health-care cost that you pay. A typical level is 15 percent. That means you pay 15 percent of each doctor visit, hospital visit, and test and the insurance pays the remaining 85 percent. Of course, that's only after you've met your deductible.

Community Health Care: The ACA provides additional funding for community health centers. They provide primary care for those on Medicaid or who cannot get health insurance, including undocumented immigrants.

Community Transformation Grants: The ACA empowers the CDC to award grants to local health and human services agencies for preventive programs. They are targeted to help people improve their lifestyles to prevent cancer, diabetes, and heart disease. In 2011, the CDC awarded $103 million and in 2012 it awarded $70 million. For more, see www.cdc.gov/nccdphp/dch/programs/communitytransformation/index.htm.

Comparative Effectiveness Research: More than half of medical treatments used by doctors have not been proven effective by research, according to a study by the Institute of Medicine, part of the National Academies. The Institute suggests conducting more cost/benefit analyses between different treatments to give doctors and patients data to make decisions on what treatments to use. The ACA authorized $1.1 billion to fund this effort. The research will be directed by a twenty-one-member Patient-Centered Outcomes Research Institute. For more, see www.healthaffairs.org/healthpolicybriefs/brief.php?brief_id=28.

Consumer Operated and Oriented Plans: The ACA created a $3.8 billion loan program for nonprofit health plans. Like any other co-op, these insurers are owned and directed by their customers. They are designed to offer low-cost insurance options. For more, see www.cms.gov/CCIIO/Resources/Fact-Sheets-and-FAQs/coop_final_rule.html.

Consumer Price Index (CPI): The nation's measurement of inflation. It's used to adjust the income qualification levels for the federal poverty level, upon which Obama-care subsidies are based.

Co-payment: A set fee you pay for each doctor or hospital visit and for each prescription. A typical co-payment is $20 for a doctor visit, $50 for a hospital visit, and $10 to $40 for each prescription. For preventive care, your co-payment is zero thanks to the ACA.

Critical Access Hospital: These are small, rural hospitals that are designed to treat common emergencies. They have twenty-five or fewer inpatient beds, keep patients for ninety-six hours or less, but must be open twenty-four hours a day, seven days a week. More complicated conditions are referred to larger, regional hospitals. They are designated as such by the US Department of Health and Human Services. Critical access hospitals receive payment from Medicare based on their actual costs, not the standard negotiated rates. That assures they receive enough to cover their costs, which tend to be higher.

Cultural Competency Training: The ACA provides scholarships and grants to train more health-care professionals to be bilingual and to understand diverse cultures. Nearly all (84 percent) of community centers and 63 percent of hospitals provide services every day to people who don't speak English very well. As a result, they are more likely to wind up back in the hospital because they didn't understand their instructions.

Death Panels: Forty percent of people surveyed believe that the ACA created death panels of government officials who decided who deserved to get coverage by federal programs like Medicare, Medicaid, and Obamacare. This was not true. It came from a misunderstanding of the ACA's proposal to allow Medicare to pay for doctor appointments for patients who wanted to discuss end-of-life care, such as do-not-resuscitate orders and living wills. The resultant uproar meant this coverage was dropped from the final bill.

Deductibles: The amount you have to pay each year in qualified medical costs before the insurance "kicks in" to cover costs. Deductibles can range anywhere from $500 a year (usually only available from company-sponsored plans) to $6,600 a year. They are annual, which means the deductible starts over January 1 of each year. Usually, the lower the deductible, the higher the premium, co-payment, or coinsurance. As health-care costs have grown, more people have opted for higher-deductible plans to keep their monthly premiums affordable. Under Obamacare, preventive care is always free, even if you haven't met your deductible.

Donut Hole: The donut hole is a gap in coverage that originally occurred in the Medicare Part D Prescription Drug plan. The gap began once you and your plan spent $2,850 a year. After that, you paid 100 percent for the drugs until you hit a $4,550 ceiling, at which point the insurance picked up its share again, usually 95 percent of the cost. The ACA subsidizes your payment in the gap. In 2010, seniors received a direct subsidy of $250; in 2011, a 50 percent discount on brand-name prescription drugs and 7 percent on generic drugs. In 2015, the donut hole started at $2,906, rising to $3,310 in 2016. Your share is reduced to 45 percent of the cost of prescription drugs, and 65 percent of generic drugs' costs. By 2020, the donut hole will be eliminated so you'll only pay 25 percent of the cost of drugs. More than eight million older Americans saved $11.5 billion because of lower prescription drug costs under the ACA. For more details about how this affects your out-of-pocket costs, see www.medicare.gov/part-d/costs/coverage-gap/part-d-coverage-gap.html.

Dual Eligible: The 9.6 million people who qualify for Medicare and have low enough incomes to qualify for Medicaid. These are the sickest and poorest people. They make up 15 percent of Medicaid beneficiaries, but 39 percent of Medicaid's cost. Similarly, they're 21 percent of the people on Medicare, but use up 36 percent of its budget. The ACA establishes two new agencies to coordinate care for these beneficiaries with a goal to reduce costs.

Emergency Medicaid: This allows undocumented immigrants, foreign students, and visitors to receive emergency medical treatment and have it covered by Medicaid. It differs by state. To give you an idea, here's New York's version: To be considered, the emergency medical condition must seriously place the patient's health in jeopardy, impair a bodily function, or damage an organ. This includes emergency labor and delivery, but not transplants or treatment of any chronic condition—even if withdrawal of Medicaid could result in death. The coverage can last for fifteen months. For more on New York's version, see www.health.ny.gov/health_care/medicaid/emergency_medical_condition_faq.htm.

Emergency Medical Treatment and Labor Act (EMTALA): This 1986 federal law forbids hospitals that accept Medicare funding to turn away any patient that arrives at the emergency room, regardless of their ability to pay or legal status. They must evaluate and stabilize the patients. Hospitals with a special facility, like a burn unit, must accept transfers of all patients. The law was passed to keep hospitals from "dumping" uninsured and poor patients onto public hospitals.

Employer Mandate: Employers with fifty or more workers must offer health insurance or pay a fine. For more information, see chapter 10.

Episode-Based Payment: The ACA authorized Medicare and insurance companies to use this method of payment to cut costs. It pays health-care providers for each "episode," such as a heart attack, stroke, or joint replacement. It replaces fee-for-service, which pays for each diagnosis, surgery, or test ordered. It saves money by giving doctors an incentive to reduce duplicate tests or diagnoses, as they try to lower their costs below the episode-based payment level.

Evidence-Based Guidelines: Analysis of insurance claims, patient records, and research is used to recommend the most successful treatments for a given diagnosis. Guidelines are also based on data analysis from insurance claims, patient records, and Medicare/Medicaid data. These guidelines are used to improve quality and reduce costs. For difficult or complex cases, doctors refer to special boards that have developed guidelines for care based on the latest research findings. For more, see www.guideline.gov.

Exchanges: Also known as health-care exchanges. These are marketplaces where you can compare different types of insurance policies that qualify under the ACA. You can find out if you're eligible for subsidies. They are either run by the state, the US Department of Health and Human Services, or a combination of both. Find out more at healthcare.gov.

Exemption: You are exempt from the ACA tax if you don't make enough to pay income taxes, were uninsured for less than three months, were in jail, or lived outside the United States. You're also exempt if you are a member of a Native American tribe, a health-care sharing ministry, or a religious sect that objects to any form of insurance. For all exemption categories, see chapter 6.

If you qualify for a hardship exemption, you can apply for low-cost catastrophic insurance. It covers hospitalization and preventive care but has a high deductible.

Federal Poverty Level: The federal poverty level is used by the US government to define who is poor. It's based on a family's annual cash income, rather than its total wealth, annual consumption, or its own assessment of well-being. The poverty level guidelines are issued each January by the Department of Health and Human Services (HHS). It's used to determine who receives federal subsidies or aid. These programs include welfare programs such as food stamps, Medicaid, and of course the ACA. For specific guidelines, see chapter 7.

Fee-for-Service: This is the traditional payment system offered by health insurance companies, Medicare, and Medicaid. With this system, doctors and other health-care providers receive a fee for each service, such as an office visit, test, surgery, or other procedure. This system is being replaced under the ACA with bundled payments, which are based on healthy outcomes.

Flexible Spending Accounts: This is a benefit offered by your insurance company. It allows you to save pretax dollars in an account that you can use throughout the year to pay for qualified health care. Historically, whatever you didn't use during the year did not roll over into the next year. The ACA has reduced the amount you can put into the account as a way to increase tax revenue and pay for other ACA benefits. However, it now allows you to roll over any excess (up to $500) into the following year.

Formulary: The list of drugs approved by your health insurance company and how much of the price is covered. It can change at any time, depending on negotiations among the insurer, the employer, and drug companies. Formularies typically include name-brand drugs that are covered by a patent, and generics, which are cheaper knock-offs that spring up when the patent wears off. You can find the formulary on your health plan's website.

Gold Plan: Insurance pays 80 percent of your health-care costs, while you pay 20 percent through your choice of deductibles, co-pays, and coinsurance rates. Most Gold plans have very low deductibles.

Grandfathered in Health Plan: Your plan may be "grandfathered in" if your plan was issued to you on or before March 23, 2010. These plans are not required to follow most of the ACA rules and so may be cheaper. However, you want to check all of their details because they may also have annual limits, lifetime limits, and not cover preventive services. In the long run, they may be more expensive than a subsidized plan bought on the exchanges. To find out, check the date you first received the plan or ask your insurance company.

Hardship Exemption: Sixteen situations where you don't have to have insurance and are exempt from the tax penalty. You can file for a hardship exemption if you were: homeless, evicted, a recipient of a shut-off notice from a utility company, a victim of domestic violence, or if you experienced one of the many other hardships. You're also exempt if your income was 138 percent or below the poverty level and your state didn't expand Medicaid. You're exempt if you filed for bankruptcy in the last six months, a fire or flood damaged your home, you're in debt due to medical expenses, or your expenses rose from caring for a sick family member. If your child was denied Medicaid or CHIP, and someone else was supposed to pay for medical support and didn't, you won't be penalized. If it turns out you were eligible for subsidies, but the insurance company didn't give them to you and so you were without insurance, you can be exempt. For more, see www.healthcare.gov/exemptions/.

Health Insurance Marketplace: This is also known as the health insurance exchange. It's where people can compare different health insurance plans, find out how much of a subsidy they might receive, and purchase insurance. They can also find out if they're eligible for Medicaid and sign up for it. The exchanges are either run by the state or the federal government. To find out more, go to HealthCare.gov.

Health Maintenance Organization (HMO): This is a type of plan where you receive all of of your primary care from one doctor, and you need a referral from him or her to see other doctors and specialists. It costs less than a preferred provider organization (PPO), but you have less choice.

Health Reimbursement Accounts: The employer contributes to an account you can use to pay for medical expenses.

Health Savings Accounts (HSA): Allows you to put pretax dollars aside to pay for medical expenses. However, you must be in a high-deductible insurance plan to use it. Whatever you don't use can be rolled over to the next year.

High-Deductible Health Insurance: According to the IRS, a high-deductible plan is one with a deductible of $1,250 per person, or $2,500 per family. Insurance companies use high-deductible plans to make sure patients "have some skin in the game." In other words, they use them to make sure policyholders don't rack up a lot of doctor bills when they aren't really sick. These plans are usually offered with health reimbursement accounts or health savings accounts to help pay for medical bills until the deductible is met. Usually, high-deductible plans have lower premiums.

Hospital-Acquired Conditions: These are medical complications that occur as a result of being in the hospital. The five most common are bedsores, blood clots from surgery, cuts, problems breathing, and infections. Others include bad interactions from medications, urinary tract infections from catheters, blood infections from drip lines, falls, pneumonia from ventilators, and thromboembolisms.

Independent Payment Advisory Board (IPAB): This board will save $3 billion by monitoring and suggesting changes to reduce Medicare's cost.

Individual Mandate: Every US citizen must get health insurance or pay a tax. This was imposed by the ACA to lower health-care and insurance costs.

In Network: A health-care provider that is in your health insurance plan's network. Your out-of-pocket cost will be lower than if you use a physician who is out of the network.

Lifetime Limit: The health insurance company only paid medical expenses up to this limit, usually $1 million to $2 million. These were banned by the ACA.

Long-Term Care Facility: These are either nursing homes or assisted living facilities that provide help for those who can't care for themselves completely.

Mandatory Budget Spending: The mandatory budget estimates the costs for US federal programs that have already been established by acts of Congress. These include Social Security, Medicare, Medicaid, food stamps, child tax credits, TANF (more commonly known as welfare), and housing assistance. Congress cannot reduce the funding for these programs without changing the authorization law that created them.

Medicaid: A health insurance program for low-income people. It was established in 1965. It is run by the states but mostly funded by the federal government. The Children's Health Insurance Program (CHIP) was added in 1997.

Medicaid Expansion: The ACA expands Medicaid to households that are 138 percent or less of the federal poverty level. For more, see chapter 7.

Medical Loss Ratio: The ACA mandates that insurance companies must spend at least 80 percent of premiums collected on benefits. For large group plans, the ratio is 85 percent. If a company doesn't meet that minimum, it must refund the difference to its enrollees. This prevents companies from spending too much on administration, advertising, or executive salaries.

Medicare: Also known as Original Medicare, this is the nation's health insurance program. It's available for seniors sixty-five and older, younger people with disabilities, and people with permanent kidney failure or ALS (amyotrophic lateral sclerosis, commonly known as Lou Gehrig's disease). You can go to any doctor that accepts Medicare, and they submit the claims for you. You have to pay a deductible, a co-payment, and coinsurance. You're automatically signed up if you enroll in Social Security before sixty-five; otherwise you have to manually sign up at the Social Security office. To apply: www.socialsecurity.gov/medicare/apply.html. For more, see medicare.gov.

Medicare Advantage: These are private insurance plans that offer Medicare Parts A, B, C, and typically Part D as well. You receive your Medicare Parts A and B from the insurance company. The federal government pays them to manage your Medicare coverage. You must sign up for Medicare Advantage to receive Part C benefits.

Medicare Part A: This covers care at hospitals, skilled nursing facilities, and nursing homes (as long as they are more than just assisted living), home health services, and hospice. It's given to everyone who's eligible (has paid Medicare payroll taxes for at least ten years). There's no premium if you're eligible. Otherwise, the premium is $425 a month. If you were not automatically enrolled, you should sign up three months before your sixty-fifth birthday, even if you're not ready to receive retirement benefits.

Medicare Part B: You have to sign up for this part of Medicare, which covers doctor visits, lab tests, surgeries, and supplies (like wheelchairs and walkers). It covers 100 percent of preventive services, like flu shots. Part B also covers clinical research, ambulance services, durable medical equipment, mental health treatment (including inpatient, outpatient, and partial hospitalization), getting a second opinion, and limited outpatient prescription drugs. Most people pay the Part B premium of $104.90 each month. Medicare Parts A and B don't cover long-term care, dental or vision care, hearing aids, or prescription or over-the-counter medicine.

Medicare Part C: This is the name for the extra benefits provided only by Medicare Advantage plans. This coverage typically includes vision, hearing, dental, and/or health and wellness programs. It costs extra above your Part B premium. The amount depends on your insurance provider.

Medicare Part D: These are prescription drug insurance plans you buy in addition to Medicare Parts A and B. You must sign up for it separately or as part of a Medicare Advantage plan.

Medigap: This is a supplemental insurance plan that you use to help cover the cost of Medicare deductibles, co-payments, and coinsurance. Unlike Medicare Advantage plans, it offers no additional benefits. You must have Medicare Parts A and B to get Medigap, but you can't have a Medicare Advantage Plan at the same time.

Obamacare: The popular name for the Affordable Care Act, which was pushed forward by President Barack Obama. It was originally only used by opponents of the ACA, who meant it to be a derogatory term. However, it was eventually adopted by President Obama himself when he said that he liked the term because he does care.

Observation Care: When doctors don't admit patients to the hospital but keep them for observation. This could be happening more often as hospitals try to avoid the ACA penalty for readmittance (see chapter 3). Observation costs are paid by Medicare Part B, which translates to higher out-of-pocket costs for you. If you're then transferred to a nursing home, Medicare won't pay the costs since you weren't officially admitted to the hospital.

Open Enrollment Period: The period of time you can sign up for health insurance through the exchanges. For coverage beginning in 2016, the enrollment period is from November 1, 2015 to January 31, 2016. Although the enrollment period has changed since 2014, it is usually around this time frame. You can use the exchanges to compare plans and review your benefits at any time throughout the year. You can also enroll for Medicaid, CHIP, or a private insurance plan at any time. Finally, you can use the exchanges if you move to a new state, marry, divorce, have a baby, or experience a big change in income.

Out-of-Network: A health-care provider who doesn't participate in your insurance network. You will probably pay more.

Out-of-Pocket Costs: This is the cost of your medical bills plus all insurance costs except premiums. It includes your deductible (what you have to meet before the insurance kicks in), co-payments (what you pay for each visit and prescription), and coinsurance (your share of health-care costs after the insurance kicks in). It doesn't apply to uncovered costs such as over-the-counter medicines, premiums, your payments to out-of-network providers, and services besides the ten essential benefits.

Out-of-Pocket Maximum: If you buy a plan on the exchange, you won't pay more than $6,600 for an individual plan or $13,200 for a family plan for 2015. This amount changes each year to keep up with inflation. Once you've paid out this amount in deductibles, coinsurance, co-payments, or similar eligible expenses, the plan pays 100 percent of the rest of qualified medical expenses. You can't count premiums, payments to non-network providers, or spending outside of the ten essential health benefits.

Platinum Plan: Your insurance company will pick up 90 percent of health-care costs. You pay 10 percent through co-pays, deductibles, and coinsurance. Most platinum plans have a zero deductible. This is a good plan if you know your medical costs will be higher than your premiums.

Poverty Level: The income levels set by the Department of Health and Human Services to define poverty. The Poverty Level is used as a basis to determine who is eligible for various federal benefits. It changes each year based on price increases. For recent updates, see "How the Poverty Level Accounts for Inflation," at http://aspe.hhs.gov/poverty/faq.cfm#CPI.

Many programs award subsidies to those with higher incomes, such as 150 percent of the federal poverty level. For a family of four, that's 1.5 x $24,250 = $36,375. For more, see "HHS 2015 Federal Poverty Guidelines," at http://aspe.hhs.gov/poverty/15poverty.cfm.

Preauthorization: Often your insurance company requires you to get authorization before you can get certain services, treatments, and medications. This is waived in an emergency.

Preexisting Condition: Any health condition diagnosis that insurance companies used to deny coverage. For more, see chapter 5.

Preferred Provider Organizations (PPO): The insurance plan that prefers you use providers within its network. Your plan will cover some of the cost if you go out of network, but it will be higher. You don't need a referral.

Premium: The amount you pay every month just to have insurance. Just like auto or homeowners insurance, you pay this even if you never make a claim. If you're usually healthy, it can be a big waste of money. However, if you incur a massive hospital bill, it will be a wise investment. Usually a lower premium means you will have a higher coinsurance, co-payment, and/or deductible.

Preventive Care: This is a very specific list of care items, specifically doctor visits and tests that are 100 percent covered under Obamacare, regardless of co-payments or deductibles. It includes screenings, annual checkups, and patient counseling to prevent illnesses, disease, or other health problems. For more, see chapter 5.

Primary Care Physician: The doctor that provides most of your medical care. He or she will refer you to specialists or the hospital when needed.

Provider Networks: The health-care providers who work with your health insurance company.

Silver Plan: Pays 70 percent of your health-care costs. You pay 30 percent overall through deductibles, co-pays, and coinsurance. You can choose the mixture. Deductibles tend to be in the $2,000 for singles/$4,000 for families range.

Skilled Nursing Facility: Also known as a nursing home, it provides skilled nursing care twenty-four hours a day. This usually includes tending to wounds, giving intravenous medicine, and providing physical or speech therapy. These facilities usually have pharmacies, medical labs, and even imaging services on-site.

Subsidies: The federal government pays all or part of your health insurance premiums if your income is 400 percent of the federal poverty level or less. For more, see chapter 7.

INDEX

W